D1263047

INHERITING MADNESS

Medicine and Society
Andrew Scull, Editor

This series examines the development of medical knowledge and psychiatric practice from historical and sociological perspectives. The books contribute to a scholarly and critical reflection on the nature and role of medicine and psychiatry in modern societies.

INHERITING MADNESS

*Professionalization and
Psychiatric Knowledge in
Nineteenth-Century France*

IAN R. DOWBIGGIN

UNIVERSITY OF CALIFORNIA PRESS
BERKELEY   LOS ANGELES   OXFORD

RC 450
.F7 D68
1991

University of California Press
Berkeley and Los Angeles, California

University of California Press, Ltd.
Oxford, England

© 1991 by
The Regents of the University of California

Library of Congress Cataloging-in-Publication Data

Dowbiggin, Ian R.
    Inheriting madness : professionalization and psychiatric
knowledge in nineteenth-century France / Ian R. Dowbiggin.
        p.   cm. — (Medicine and society)
    Includes bibliographical references.
    ISBN 0-520-06937-4
    1. Psychiatry—France—History—19th century.
2. Mental illness—France—History—19th century.
    I. Title.   II. Series.
    RC450.F7D68   1991
    616.89′00944′09034—dc20   90-10914
                                                        CIP

Printed in the United States of America
1   2   3   4   5   6   7   8   9

The paper used in this publication meets the minimum
requirements of American National Standard for Information
Sciences—Permanence of Paper for Printed Library Materials,
ANSI Z39.48–1984. ♾

To Terry and her love of the world of ideas

Contents

Acknowledgments

This book began as a doctoral dissertation at the University of Rochester, which generously supported my research overseas. Two scholars in particular deserve my deepest thanks. William J. McGrath drew often from his sophisticated understanding of intellectual history to help me refine my approach to the topic I had chosen. Theodore M. Brown's sensitivity to the history of professional knowledge also proved invaluable when I undertook to explain why nineteenth-century French psychiatrists thought the way they did. Others whose conversation and writings I have enjoyed during the preparation of this book include Edward M. Brown, William F. Bynum, Toby Gelfand, Jan Goldstein, George Grinnell, Steve Kunitz, Christopher Lasch, Mark Micale, Randy Schiffer, Sam Shortt, Larry Stewart, Corinne Sutter, and Nancy Tomes. While few of them would agree with all my conclusions, each has influenced my thinking and I owe them all a considerable intellectual debt. The same and more can be said for Andrew Scull, whose patience and encouragement were critical to the process of revising the dissertation manuscript for publication. Thanks also go to Tammy Johnston, who typed the revisions promptly and efficiently, and to Mary Lamprech and Ilene O'Malley of the University of California Press for their editorial contributions.

But above all, I wish to thank my wife, Christine. Without her love and support this book would have been impossible.

Parts of this book have appeared previously in the following publications: "Degeneration and Hereditarianism in French Mental Medicine, 1840–1890: Psychiatric Theory as Ideological Adaptation," in *The Anatomy of Madness: Essays in the History of Psychiatry*, 2 vols., ed. W. F. Bynum, Roy Porter, and Michael Shepherd (London: Tavistock, 1985), 1:188–232; "French Psychiatry, Hereditarianism, and Professional Legitimacy, 1840–1900," in *Research in Law, Deviance and Social Control*, 10 vols., ed. Andrew T. Scull and Steven Spitzer (Greenwich, Conn.: JAI Press, 1985), 7:135–65; "French Psychiatric Attitudes Towards the Dangers Posed by the Insane, ca. 1870," in Scull and Spitzer, eds. (1988), 9:87–111; "French Psychiatry and the Search for a Professional Identity: The *Société médico-psychologique*, 1840–1870," *Bulletin of the History of Medicine* 63 (1989):331–55. I would like to thank the publishers for their permission to reproduce copyrighted material.

Introduction

If cancer is arguably the disease of the twentieth century, then it is
equally arguable that mental illness was the disease of the nineteenth century. Or so thought the French republican deputy Léon
Gambetta. Speaking before the *Corps législatif* on 21 March 1870,
Gambetta claimed that public concern over the rising number of
hospitalized lunatics and the incapacity of asylum psychiatrists to
tame insanity was mounting "to the point," he stressed, "where
madness seems to be the disease of the century."[1] Gambetta may
not have been far wrong. Like cancer in this century,[2] mental illness in the nineteenth century sparked public fear and revulsion
and symbolized mystery and the limits of human power. Physicians
knew little about what caused it, what its ultimate nature was, or
how to cure it, but they still insisted that the best interests of those
who suffered from it were served by early diagnosis by members of
organized medicine. Psychiatrists accused nonmedical people who
tried to treat it of quackery and ignorance. They argued that mental
disease was caused neither by sin nor by personal moral failure, yet
they themselves relied on naturalist explanations that ultimately
blamed individual life-style for mental illness. These and other
contradictions in medical thinking about madness did not escape
the notice of people like Gambetta, who concluded that psychiatrists posed a grave threat to public health, self-reliance, and individual freedom.

No theory of mental disease enjoyed as much popularity in the
nineteenth century as that of mental degeneracy.[3] According to this
theory certain families suffered a steady though not necessarily irre-

versible hereditary deterioration over the course of four generations. These families customarily displayed symptoms such as moral
depravity, mania, mental retardation, and sterility. Physicians ascribed a variety of causes to degeneracy, including alcoholism, immorality, poor diet, and unhealthy domestic and occupational conditions. However, the principal cause of degeneracy that physicians
cited was heredity. Indeed, so strong was the tendency of French
mental doctors to regard heredity as a causal factor that they commonly considered mental degeneracy to be simply hereditary
weakness, a belief reinforced by the absence (until the end of the
nineteenth century) of any clear distinction between innate and
acquired characteristics. Thus degeneracy and heredity were virtually synonymous for many French psychiatrists—or "alienists," as
they liked to call themselves.[4]

The doctrine of hereditary degeneracy was first formulated in the
1850s. It drew increasing attention for the next twenty-five years
and enjoyed its greatest popularity in the 1880s and 1890s. After
1900 its popularity waned, yet for the physician Georges Genil-
Perrin, a positivist, early twentieth-century French psychiatrist, its
rise to prominence represented a progressive step in the early history of psychiatry. With the notion of hereditarianism, he argued,
mental medicine liberated itself from "metaphysics" and theology
and took its place among the other "positive" sciences. As a result,
he also argued, psychiatry's fortunes improved considerably, a process smoothed by the fact that degeneracy theory enjoyed widespread public favor.[5]

It is somewhat surprising, then, that there has been no historically comprehensive account since Genil-Perrin's of this major
chapter of psychiatry's intellectual past.[6] This study is intended to
fill this gap. Like Genil-Perrin, I shall describe the origins and the
evolution of hereditarianism from roughly the mid-1800s to the fin
de siècle period, with particular attention to the history of degeneracy theory. Unlike Genil-Perrin, who predictably interpreted
matters from the perspective of an early twentieth-century psychiatrist proud of his profession's accomplishments, I shall show that
his positivist interpretation does not do justice to the historical reality of nineteenth-century asylum medicine. Genil-Perrin believed that the "liberation" of psychiatry from "metaphysics" and
theology was part of a simultaneous improvement in psychiatric

knowledge. Yet after over 150 years of pathoanatomical, biochemical, and physiological research, the same nagging obscurities characterize the domain of mental medicine: somatic pathology is still unclear; "etiology remains speculative, pathogenesis largely obscure, classification predominantly symptomatic and hence arbitrary and possibly ephemeral; physical treatments are empirical and subject to fashion, and psychotherapies still only in their infancy and doctrinaire."[7] In 1975 a leading American psychiatrist agreed, stating that mental medicine had yet to reach "an understanding of the basic causes and mechanisms" of psychosis and neurosis.[8] If, then, psychiatry's fortunes rose between 1850 and 1900 by virtue of its adoption of degeneracy theory, its progress was not based on a precise understanding of insanity or improvements in the treatment of madness; its shifting status as a medical specialty derived instead from a complex conjuncture of sociopolitical, cultural, and professional circumstances.

What led to the shift toward degeneracy theory? The answer is in part related to the emergence of French mental medicine in the middle third of the nineteenth century as a distinct medical specialty. In the preceding two hundred years insanity had been regarded as a form of social deviance. The insane were housed with beggars, abandoned children, criminals, and prostitutes in general hospitals, created by royal edict in 1662 as a combination workhouse, prison, old people's home, orphanage, and reformatory. Michel Foucault has described the creation of the general hospitals throughout France as "the great confinement" because they constituted an institutional answer to the problems of social deviance in the seventeenth and eighteenth centuries.[9] By the nineteenth century the insane were distributed randomly throughout the general hospitals, prisons, poorhouses, and religious hospices of each *département*. In Paris the medical profession finally began to assume custodial responsibility for the mad during the Empire (1804–1815) and Restoration (1815–1830), yet it was not until the July Monarchy (1830–1848) that doctors outside Paris took a serious interest in the institutionalized insane. Even in early nineteenth-century Montpellier—whose school of medicine was second only to that of Paris in prestige—doctors had tended to ignore the institutionalized lunatics of the city until a pupil of the celebrated psychiatrist J. E. D. Esquirol arrived in 1821 to refurbish the existing insane asylum in accord with Philippe Pinel's "moral treatment."[10] Moral treatment, a form of therapy based on a faith in the healing powers of nature and a rejection of drugs and physical restraint, held that mentally ill persons could regain their senses most quickly if removed from their everyday environment and placed in institutions specially designed to soothe their feelings and protect them from upsetting stimuli. Both because it appeared to be a benevolent way of treating madness and because it endorsed institutional isolation for people who threatened social order, moral treatment encouraged French legislators to pass the Law of 30 June 1838. This law establishing the guidelines for the national system of public asylums accelerated medical involvement in the custodial care of the insane and also marked the beginnings of the psychiatric profession as a corps of state functionaries entrusted with the institutional study and cure of mental disease.

Psychiatry's future looked promising by 1840. Physicians attracted to the study of lunacy willingly accepted the challenge to eliminate the punitive and often barbaric methods that previous custodians of the mad had employed. However, there were clouds on the horizon. With the decline of pathological explanations based on localized structural damage to the body's organs and the rise of medical theories emphasizing functional processes, many doctors began to question their belief that madness had a physical basis. This questioning was potentially calamitous for alienists. If madness and its mood disorders were primarily psychological phenomena without discernible physical lesions, then there was no rationale for exclusively medical intervention in cases of mental derangement nor for claiming that alienists rather than academic psychologists were uniquely qualified to distinguish a morbid mental state from genius or simple eccentricity. These psychiatric difficulties were compounded by the rise in the 1860s of a predominantly lay movement that questioned the need for large, medically supervised asylums as the principal form of public assistance to the insane. These factors combined with a persistent popular and juridical suspicion of psychiatric views on criminal responsibility to convince asylum physicians of the need for a cognitive model of pathology to legitimize their diagnostic, therapeutic, and social approaches to madness.

Philosophic and sociopolitical considerations exacerbated psychiatry's troubles. Throughout the century French scholars wrote extensively on the relationship of body to mind. As physicians of mental medicine, psychiatrists were unavoidably implicated in this debate, which many entered in the middle third of the nineteenth century. Some adopted the physiological argument that even the highest mental functions were governed by the natural laws that governed organized matter; others took the more orthodox spiritualist position that these functions were ultimately independent of organic processes. As a result, rifts developed within the profession. When the Catholic reaction of the Second Empire (1852–1870) made the mind-body debate all the more germane, these rifts became a source of embarrassment for psychiatrists because they highlighted fundamental differences of opinion within a group of physicians who were adamantly trying to convince others that they constituted a learned profession united by a scientific body of knowledge. Clericalist attacks during the Second Empire on those who cultivated secular approaches to knowledge also disquieted psychiatrists whose medical training automatically made them suspicious to Catholic officials. Psychiatric anxieties about the possibility of persecution only began to diminish with the end of the monarchical threat to the Third Republic in 1877 and the rise to power of politicians sympathetic to the ideology of naturalist science. By then, however, psychiatrists had developed a wary attitude toward their political and social environment. They came to believe that their claims to expertise were threatened by popular forces inimical to their naturalist and rationalist world view.

I shall contend that it was this profound sense of defensiveness and insecurity that led to the widespread psychiatric acceptance of degeneracy theory in the final third of the nineteenth century. Hereditary degeneracy theory provided asylum physicians with a unitary concept that encompassed pathological behavior and affect in psychological, biological, and social terms.[11] It was remarkably eclectic and free-ranging in scope: because it incorporated so many aspects of behavioral and biological sciences under one rubric, it was ideal for disguising the inconsistencies and anomalies of psychiatric knowledge while strengthening physicians' claim to expertise. As a principle for classifying mental diseases, the theory enabled psychiatric clinicians to depict themselves as scientific because it was seemingly based on the etiological notion that there was a physical cause of insanity: heredity. Degeneracy theory could claim to be both

scientific and somatic; it led to treatments that were moral and were conveyed as such; and it brought the phenomenon of madness into contact with the social world. . . . Above all, it was comprehensible. Its advocates and its converts promised to provide at a stroke solutions to the mysteries of character, personality, talent or the lack of it, crime, and madness.[12]

Just as important, degeneracy theory and the hereditarianism it spawned constituted an intellectual model that in France, as in nineteenth-century America, imposed "a consoling order upon a continually shifting reality."[13] These features of degeneracy theory enabled the psychiatric community to gain the turn-of-the-century confidence and relative unity that Genil-Perrin observed.

Yet psychiatrists did not conjure up hereditarian ideas out of nowhere. Hereditarian theory was used in much of contemporaneous French medicine, especially with respect to constitutional and chronic diseases; it corresponded to the prevailing interest in evolutionary biology and anthropology and blended nicely with the more general attitudes toward crime, psychology, and politics pervading French culture near the end of the century. Thus the nineteenth-century French psychiatric fondness for the theory of hereditary degeneracy largely derived from the attempt to solve professional difficulties by adopting a popular biomedical, philosophic, and cultural concept.[14] Intellectual accomodation played at least as large a role in the development of French psychiatry between 1840 and 1900 as did intellectual struggle. The way in which psychiatry developed from an uncertain medical specialty linked to political heterodoxy to a generally accredited medical practice can best be understood in the context of the social and scientific changes in France during the same period.

One organization in particular played a crucial role in this historical process: the Paris-based Société médico-psychologique. Its journal, the *Annales médico-psychologiques*, was launched in 1843, the first exclusively psychiatric journal in France. The Société itself was founded in 1852, after an attempt to found such an organization in 1848 had failed, and soon boasted the membership of virtually all the prominent figures in French psychiatry. The *Annales médico-*

psychologiques quickly became the forum for France's leading alienists and featured articles on a wide range of issues dealing with psychopathology. The minutes of the Société's meetings, published in the *Annales*, provide a revealing look at many of the physicians who staffed the asylums of France. The *Annales* served as the mouthpiece for the Société and consequently for the entire community of French psychiatrists. No other contemporary association or journal could claim the allegiance of so many preeminent medical men.[15] Therefore, it was an excellent barometer of French psychiatric attitudes toward French society, general medicine, and the subgroups that made up the psychiatric profession itself.

The Société médico-psychologique is the focus for this study. No other treatment of nineteenth-century French psychiatry has been based on an organization so clearly representative of French alienism as the Société médico-psychologique.[16] Biographical material pertaining to some of the Société's central figures provides insight into how theories of insanity were influenced by professional and political motives. Although I stress external factors and their impact on psychiatric thinking, I do not wish to suggest that personal motives are inconsequential. As one historian has written:

Rejecting deterministic interpretations of the sociology of knowledge, I nevertheless believe that things like social structures, institutional constraints, and professional role models more or less strongly bias someone working within their sphere of influence to hold or not to hold certain basic attitudes towards knowledge. Yet in the final analysis it is the individual who, consciously or unconsciously, chooses from among the available alternatives in dealing with the particular problems he faces. . . . [S]ocial forces do not translate in some magical or inexorable way into attitudes held. Rather, it is the negotiating individual who must lie at the epistemological center of any nondeterministic sociology of knowledge. Somehow our notions of the relevance of the social context of scientific activity, and hence our theories about that nexus, must be rich enough to allow for both widespread attitudinal conformity and individual variance.[17]

The experience of French psychiatry in the nineteenth century is an important chapter in the relatively new field of the history of the professions.[18] I shall use S. E. D. Shortt's definition of professionalization as "a process by which a heterogeneous collection of individuals is gradually recognized, by both themselves and other members of society, as constituting a relatively homogeneous and distinct occupational group."[19] Professionalization entails the process whereby occupational groups seek to sharpen the boundaries between themselves and other groups through special licensing and standardized training, to restrict the practice of specific skills to certain occupational groups, and to augment the services the groups provide to society. All these elements of professionalization apply to nineteenth-century psychiatry. Psychiatrists discovered early in the century that as physicians they had been granted important privileges in the diagnosis and treatment of madness, even though they had displayed no conclusive competence in either capacity. The professional history of psychiatry in France for the rest of the century is essentially the story of how physicians developed forms of knowledge that obscured this embarrassing gap between social power and technical effectiveness. This endeavor was crucial not just for the defense of psychiatric prerogatives but also for the expansion of medicine's authority into areas of practice dominated by lay men and women.

The history of psychiatric knowledge also reflects the social marginality of asylum physicians. While the history of the professions of western Europe since the French Revolution may be a success story, success for French physicians was not easily achieved.[20] Although they had been granted a medical monopoly by Napoleon in 1803, most doctors, "continued to view themselves as an unappreciated and insufficiently rewarded occupational group within French society" until the end of the century.[21] As members of the medical profession, then, alienists were part of a socially marginal group; and as members of a barely accredited branch of medicine, they were "marginal twice over."[22] Professionalization was intended to mitigate the effects of marginality, and the construction of a body of knowledge such as degeneracy theory played a critical role in this process. By depicting themselves as proponents of the most up-to-date ideas of biological science, psychiatrists could uphold their claims to specialized expertise and gain the approval of powerful social groups whose interests were safeguarded by asylum alienists.[23] Government policy makers and the ruling middle class in France were receptive to appeals to the moral influence of science, and psychiatric support for hereditarian concepts like degeneracy theory convinced them that alienists were the professionals most capable of identifying and treating the pressing psychological problems bred of industrialization and social dislocation.[24] Thus, psychiatric thinking mirrored the concerns of France's ruling elite. Indeed, it did more; it naturalized class divisions and reinforced the social organization of acceptable forms of knowledge.[25]

My interpretation of French psychiatric ideas between the last years of the July Monarchy and World War I stresses the ways in which the alienists of the Société médico-psychologique tried to come to terms with the shifting political and cultural forces that tended to isolate psychiatrists as a professional group. In particular, the antipsychiatric press campaign of the 1860s prompted alienists to mobilize to cover psychiatry's vulnerable flanks while also encroaching upon spheres of authority enjoyed by priests, nuns, lawyers, and lay scholars. By the 1870s the psychiatric community was eager to adopt a clinical model of mental pathology that would assure other doctors and the state that alienists possessed special knowledge that proved the biological reality of mental disease and authorized psychiatrists to "refer simultaneously to the experienced mental state and its underlying physiological counterpart."[26] The theory of mental degeneracy was ideal as a model of pathology because it translated cultural and scientific themes into a neutral idiom while justifying the socially utilitarian role of the asylum doctor. Psychiatric theory in late nineteenth-century France was intended to stem the alienation of alienists, increase their acceptance as expert professionals, and disassociate them from a past characterized by wrangling, failed therapies, public hostility, and political heterodoxy.

My interpretation generally agrees with Jan Goldstein's in *Console and Classify* (1987). Goldstein maintains that the history of French psychiatric ideas such as hysteria and monomania demonstrates that from the beginning to the end of the century French alienists were engaged in a "bid for power through psychiatric knowledge," a project to expand the professional authority of psychiatry through the pursuit of secular and anticlerical goals.[27] There was also an anticlerical element in degeneracy theory because its characterization of madness as a biophysical phenomenon authorized alienists to override the religious orders who competed with medicine for control of mental hospitals.

However, anticlericalism was not the only important element of

psychiatric theory in nineteenth-century France. Goldstein mini-
mizes or overlooks the significance of factors that are emphasized
here—the revival of "moral treatment" in the 1840s, the physicalist
orientation of mental medicine, the role of the Société médico-
psychologique, the antipsychiatric movement of the 1860s, the conflict between alienism and academic psychology, tensions between
psychiatry and mainstream medicine, and the rise of hereditarianism and degeneracy theory between 1850 and 1914. These factors
were crucial because they compelled alienists to reassess their relations with the state, the public, other doctors, and other professionals.

Intent on establishing the proposition that only alienists were
capable of diagnosing and treating insanity, psychiatrists in the late
nineteenth century were also determined to cultivate an image of
political disinterest and neutral expertise. This attitude to a large
extent resulted from the alienists' difficulties adjusting to the shifting political winds of France from 1815 to 1871. By posing as specialists with unique insights into matters relating to social policy,
they hoped that their services would appear to be indispensable to
a state increasingly obsessed with class friction, crime, and the
defense of the family. True to the positivist notion that class conflict was ultimately regressive and stemmed from mass ignorance,
alienists tended to view themselves less as ideologues and more as
scientifically trained, clinically experienced civil servants who practiced their craft in public institutions. It was in this sense that
French alienists sought to professionalize in the period preceding
World War I. The politics of social defense overshadowed anticlericalism in the medical "bid for power through psychiatric knowledge."

Chapter One

The State of Psychiatric Practice and Knowledge in the Nineteenth Century

In its efforts to improve its professional standing in the early nineteenth century, French psychiatry encountered two major difficulties. In 1838 the French state gave alienists important privileges to treat the insane in public asylums. Yet at roughly the same time, the growing failure of psychiatrists to cure their patients under the conditions of hospital medicine was becoming glaringly obvious. This therapeutic failure placed great pressure on psychiatrists to demonstrate their special knowledge of insanity's causes, symptoms, and underlying organic pathology, and here too their shortcomings were evident. The stakes for psychiatrists were high because unless they could prove they possessed unequaled knowledge of mental illness there was the danger that the state would revoke some or all of their privileges and transfer them to the Catholic orders, who still participated in the treatment of psychological disorders. Similarly, psychiatrists knew that as insanity's somatic pathology became increasingly problematic, the gap between them and their colleagues in general medicine would widen. One of the initial steps physicians took to address these problems was the founding of the *Annales médico-psychologiques* in 1843, the first psychiatric journal in France. The early issues of the *Annales* mirrored the intellectual heterodoxy of psychiatry at midcentury and its eagerness to find answers to its practical and cognitive dilemmas.

Psychiatric Practice in the
Nineteenth Century

Although the public asylums provided employment opportunities
for aspiring psychiatrists, alienists found little solace in carrying
out their duties as asylum physicians. Despite the improvements
made since the eighteenth century and the perfunctory testimonials to the humanitarian reforms instituted by men such as Philippe
Pinel (1745–1826) and J. E. D. Esquirol (1772–1840), the acknowledged pioneers of nineteenth-century French psychiatry, conditions within mental hospitals remained deplorable throughout
most of the century. These conditions, the difficulties of the nas-
cent profession, and the exceedingly low prestige accorded "mad-
doctors" combined to make the psychiatrist's lot a poor one.

The state of psychiatry in the middle third of the nineteenth
century depended to a large extent on the state of French medicine
as a whole. Unfortunately for alienists, all was not well within the
medical community. The Law of 19 Ventôse Year XI (10 March
1803), which followed the suppression of the medical faculties and
the Société royal de médecine during the Revolution, reorganized
the profession by creating the titles of doctor of medicine or surgery
and health officer (*officier de santé*). The law also limited the practice of medicine by establishing a uniform national licensing system.
Yet the existence of health officers, who required simpler training,
increasingly rankled full-fledged doctors and government officials,
who resented the competition the health officers represented. In
1845 they took steps to encourage legislation against the health
officers, holding a national medical congress with Comte de Salvandy, the minister of education, in attendance. The congress
wholeheartedly endorsed improved standards of training, the aboli-
tion of health officers, and the establishment of local councils of
doctors to direct judicial authorities to combat the charlatanism of
rural quacks. When Salvandy presented his reform bill to the Chamber of Peers in 1847 he encountered stiff opposition from liberals and
Catholics who objected to the proposal to place all medical education under control of the state. Many Catholics also wished to protect the medical activities of the religious orders, whose conflict with
official physicians was "after the role of the *officiers de santé*, the
most hotly disputed issue in the nineteenth-century debates on
medical practice."[1] The 1848 revolution brought an end to Sal-

vandy's efforts to introduce reform legislation. Many French doctors had in any case been dissatisfied with his project because the proposed reforms did not satisfy their call for a greater role in the state system of medical education.[2] The medical profession's dissatisfaction with the country's medical system persisted, yet the position of health officer was not abolished until 1892.

Psychiatrists also had to face the problem of overcrowding within the medical profession at midcentury. Like other middle-class professions in western Europe between 1815 and 1848,[3] medicine suffered from the discrepancy between demand for professional services and enrollment in professional schools. If not all areas of France were saturated with doctors, Paris certainly was, with only 3 percent of the national population and 13 percent of all doctors. The result was bitter competition for patients and for salaried medical posts in hospitals. It is little wonder that the author of a popular book on career possibilities for young Frenchmen saw medicine in 1842 as a relatively poor choice because of the "long and difficult studies," lack of independence, poor salary, and public disrespect.[4] The difficulties of making a living at medicine combined with physicians' individualism, patriotism, secularism, and democratic sentiments to make many doctors impatient with the established order and supportive of the 1848 revolution.[5] An indication of medical dissatisfaction with the government of Louis Philippe was the large number of physicians who served in political and administrative posts during the Second Republic (1848–1851).

Physicians' dissatisfaction with the status quo in 1848 also helps to explain why unorthodox medical therapies such as mesmerism and homeopathy flourished at midcentury.[6] Ambitious and imaginative young physicians eager to attract patients were more willing to experiment with different therapeutic techniques than established doctors were. Orthodox medicine was alarmed that the government appeared reluctant to stamp out these alleged forms of charlatanism. However, even with a "well-developed system of medical police" local administrations could do little to enforce professional control over medical care.[7] The reasons were not hard to find. Throughout almost the entire century, the medical profession competed with a strong and widespread tradition of popular healing. Licensed doctors were usually thought to be costly and insensitive. Because of public disregard for official titles and because the standard medical education ignored many aspects of physical and

mental health, popular healers would always be in demand.[8]
Equally galling to licensed doctors was the heavy annual tax that
they paid for the privilege of practicing medicine, a tax popular
healers did not pay.[9]

Thus, although the Ventôse law of 1803 had given French doctors what was later considered to be "the first 'modern' professional
monopoly—at the time probably the tightest de jure monopoly in
the world"[10]—physicians continued to complain that the law was a
poorly designed stopgap measure whose enforcement was erratic
and which did little to solve the persistent problems of public mis-
trust and charlatanism. By the end of the century the public image
of the doctor had improved. Nonetheless, the "vast majority of doctors" thought they were grossly underpaid and unappreciated.[11]
Moreover, their guaranteed monopoly fostered little professional
cohesiveness.[12] A French medical association was not launched
until 1858, and it never attained the influence or representative
character of its American counterpart, founded in 1846.[13] If French
medicine benefited from what foreigners perceived to be the strict-
est legislation concerning the policing of medical care, it was
equally clear that its practitioners were a generally disgruntled,
restless, divided, and insecure group.

Psychiatry was one of the least attractive specialties within medicine for an aspiring young physician. In 1843, according to the
alienist Jules Baillarger (1809–1890), there were some twenty-five
to thirty doctors in Paris who worked in public or private asylums.
He calculated that outside the capital there were three times that
many who practised medicine in mental hospitals. Of this group,
the vast majority were from the middle and upper ranks of the
bourgeoisie and came from the northeast region of the country.[14]
Because they were preoccupied with administrative duties, most
public asylum alienists had no time for private practice; this was
increasingly true as the century wore on.[15] Psychiatry also was the
lowest paid medical specialty in 1848.[16] Moreover, psychiatrists
were part of the glut of doctors in France at midcentury, which
made competition for jobs fierce and exacerbated the rivalries
within the psychiatric community.[17]

Restricted for the most part to their hospitals, alienists discovered one outlet for demonstrating their expertise. This was provided by articles 43 and 44 of the Napoleonic Code of criminal
procedure, which stipulated that doctors could be called into courts

of law to testify in matters relating to the mental state of the accused and to autopsical evidence. However, doctors encountered strong opposition from both the French magistracy and public prosecutors, who tended to hold a low opinion of such testimony. Although psychiatry did make substantial inroads into legal medicine by the end of the century, this progress was not even; indeed, matters seemed to have reached a stalemate by the 1850s. Early in that decade psychiatrists debated the validity of the monomania defense, which alienists had used in the previous thirty years to explain how a person could have committed a horrendous act, such as murder, under the influence of an involuntary impulse while appearing to be rational in all other respects. The widespread alienist rejection of the concept of monomania in the fifties was influenced by the loss of credibility monomania had suffered in the eyes of French legal experts.[18] By midcentury the fortunes of alienists as medicolegal authorities had received a setback because judges and lawyers generally distrusted the psychiatric argument that insanity could diminish criminal responsibility.

Within the asylums the situation was equally dissatisfying. By midcentury there was no way an asylum doctor could ignore publicly the insalubrious surroundings in which he had to work. In the 1790s Pinel had managed to introduce some changes in the Parisian hospitals housing the insane, such as Salpêtrière and Bicêtre, where the chains had been removed from the inmates and physical violence against them drastically reduced. At the same time Pinel advocated much more thorough supervision and discipline of patients within the hospital. In 1796 a third mental hospital had been built in the Parisian suburb of Charenton along the reformist lines proposed by Pinel. In 1838 the government of Louis Philippe had responded to medical pressure and passed the law that established the legal guidelines for admission to a public asylum and set up the national system of mental institutions. Yet beyond these encouraging steps, conditions changed little and slowly, especially outside Paris.[19] Doubtless conditions in the private asylums such as psychiatrist Alexandre Brierre de Boismont's *maison de santé* in Paris, Emile Blanche's in Passy, and Jules Baillarger's and Jacques Moreau's at Ivry, which catered to the rich and middle classes, were much better. But after 1838 it was the public asylums housing the insane of the pauper classes that offered the best employment opportunities and attracted the majority of alienists; most private

asylum psychiatrists also worked in the public asylums. The
Auxerre asylum was not unusual:

The slick humid paving of the courtyards had the grave inconvenience
of chilling the lower limbs and consequently of promoting brain congestion; mephitic exhalations rising from holes dug in the ground to bury
refuse constituted a permanent source of infection . . . ; in a word, the
interior appearance of the building was more likely to arouse fear and
madness than to produce a favorable effect upon the patients' moral
state. . . .

The damp compartments—badly constructed, poorly lighted, and almost devoid of furniture—totaled *fifty-six*; yet that number must have
been considered insufficient, since *twenty-two* more were being built and
the grounds had been laid out so as to make the construction of *twenty-two*
others feasible in the future. The fifty-six compartments existing in 1839,
when the hospital housed no more than fifty madmen, were all occupied
at night, and most of them during the day as well.

There were only three bathtubs, carved of stone and fixed into the
walls, and one of them, with a shower attachment, was located in a dark
cubicle and was a real source of terror for the wretches brought there; it
was therefore physically impossible to make use of the one therapy—
baths—that is specifically recommended by physicians who have specialized in the study and treatment of mental illnesses. . . .

The inadequate dormitories were badly laid out and always open; there
was a total lack of water—in summer, at any rate—which meant that it
had to be fetched from the river; there was no laundry in the establishment, no drying room. . . . Instead of being separated into distinct categories, the patients were intermingled and mixed in such a way that epileptics would strike terror in those of their companions in misfortune who
were prey to mania or melancholy, or who were recuperating. Many of
them were constantly shut up in their compartments and as a result were
in such a frantic state that no one was allowed to approach them. . . .

Routine and wearisome, life within the institution was completely un-
coordinated; the patients generally went to bed too early; they awoke at all
hours; and their surveillance was quite poor, since it lacked above all a
purpose that could transform it into a powerful tool of healing. . . .

. . . Under such conditions, and affected by such distressing influences, the insane did not improve but, instead, rapidly reached a state of
dementia and eventually became *incurable* or else so frantic that it was
dangerous to approach them.[20]

Indeed, in some provincial hospitals conditions were even worse, as is evident from Esquirol's 1818 report on the treatment of the insane in French institutions.[21]

Conditions had improved little by 1860. Henri Girard de Cailleux (1814–1884), the inspector-general of the insane for the Seine *département*, wrote in 1861 that the overcrowding at Bicêtre and Salpêtrière had compelled administrators to transfer some patients to provincial asylums. However, by transferring these patients Girard became aware of the deplorable living conditions in many provincial mental hospitals. He discovered that equally severe overcrowding awaited them, as well as excessive use of physical restraint, inadequate clothing and diet, a higher mortality rate than among patients in Paris hospitals, exploitative labor, and the random mixing of violent, agitated, and quiet lunatics. He was also appalled to find that many inmates of provincial asylums were strapped to their beds in highly uncomfortable and literally tortuous poses.[22]

The alienist B. A. Morel (1809–1873) was hardly exaggerating, then, when he declared in 1868 that all French public asylums were in a state of "chaos, in which all the forms of intellectual degradation accumulate pell-mell, without profit to the sick or the doctors whose entire time is absorbed by writing monthly reports of the nine hundred patients they have to treat."[23] In such a state of affairs, Alexandre Brierre de Boismont (1797–1881) alleged, physicians in public asylums had no time to take the histories of individual patients and thus could not hope to acquire the personal information about their charges or to gain the insights into the etiology of insanity that private asylum doctors could.[24] The result of these dissatisfying circumstances was that the mental hospital grew to have less and less in common with ordinary hospitals. One physician complained in 1865 that life in the asylum constituted an "abnormal" situation for the insane, an environment in which physicians confined their patients for extended periods whether or not they were incurable or dangerous to society.[25] The complaint that asylums were highly inappropriate settings for healing and studying the insane was a familiar and valid refrain by the 1860s.

These conditions continued because of the reluctance of government to implement fully the asylum system reform law of 1838. That law had recommended that each *département* build special hospitals for the insane,[26] but by 1840 there were only seven asylums in France that exclusively received psychotic patients.[27] By 1852 only seven new asylums had opened, and of these only three were completely new structures, the others having been built onto existing hospitals.[28] In the Paris region, the first completely new asylum was not opened until 1867, even though the population of Paris had almost doubled since the last hospital for the insane had been built at the beginning of the nineteenth century.[29] The dramatic overcrowding had predictable effects on institutional sanitation and hygiene.[30]

Moreover, it was evident by midcentury that the majority of inmates were incurably and chronically ill,[31] a condition encouraged by the high percentage of senile and infirm individuals who still found their way into the asylums. The doctors who prepared the report on the national asylum system in 1874 pointed to the willingness of families to have their elderly or insane members institutionalized at the government's expense; in the case of psychotics, internment usually occurred long after the illness had passed from the acute to the chronic stage and the possibility of cure had vanished.[32] "The large number of aged persons" in mental hospitals, the authors added, belonged in regular hospitals and not in insane asylums.[33]

The data bear out these impressions. A surprisingly high percentage of the asylum population were patients with congenital or senile mental debility. For all French public asylum admissions in 1874, the mentally retarded of both sexes totalled 5.9 percent.[34] The percentages were higher for Paris: between 1872 and 1885, 14 percent of all male and 19 percent of all female involuntary admissions—that is, those sequestered by authority of the Parisian prefecture of police—were classed as suffering from a "senile cerebral state."[35] At Sainte-Anne, one of the capital's new asylums built in the late 1860s, twenty-four men and fifty-one women—or 13 percent of a total population of 560—were diagnosed in 1874 as suffering from senile dementia.[36]

These statistics assume even greater importance when other categories of the hospitalized population are taken into consideration. For example, there were large numbers of institutionalized patients afflicted with incurable insanity from syphilis. The rate was as high as 14.5 percent for all French public asylum admissions in 1874 and an imposing 29.2 percent for the Charenton hospital with its mostly middle-class clientele.[37] Twenty-five years earlier Baillarger had

estimated that general paresis, a condition due to syphilitic infection, characterized one-fifth and sometimes one-fourth of the cases
in a typical psychiatric establishment.[38]

Alcoholism was also rampant: among the thirty-two thousand admissions of both sexes to Paris public asylums between 1872 and
1885, 28 percent of all males were diagnosed as alcoholic.[39] At
Sainte-Anne the percentage of male alcoholics among all admissions
fluctuated from a high of 48 percent in May of 1871 to 29.88 percent
in the following month, although the figure stabilized at roughly 30
percent in the early 1880s.[40] Because the alcoholic's institutionalization ordinarily occurred after the onset of delirium tremens—as
was the case with the heroine's husband in Zola's *L'Assomoir*—
alcoholism confronted doctors with yet another irreversible illness.[41]

It is hardly surprising that the cure rate in psychiatry was low.
The steady and considerable infiltration of asylums by incurable
patients coincided with a drop in the proportion of cures to admissions in all French asylums from 27.9 percent in 1864 to 24.8 percent in 1874, despite the putative improvement in the treatment of
the insane and the construction of more modern hospitals during
the same period. The argument that if the incurable patients were
excluded from the calculation of the cure rate, the cure rate would
rise to close to 40 percent was doubtless attractive to alienists but
remained unproven.[42]

Equally distressing to psychiatrists was the low opinion people
had of them. Although some physicians noted increased public confidence in the asylum physician by the end of the century,[43] other
evidence had less positive implications. Physicians in general had a
poor reputation at midcentury.[44] Alienists in particular were dis-
tressed by the popular custom of seeking out nonmedical healers,
especially priests, to treat nervous and mental disorders. Most
French families, particularly in rural areas, turned to the sacra-
ments of the Church when members suffered from paralytic, nervous, or psychotic affections.[45] When they did minister to the
insane, alienists were never quite free of the stigma attached to
treating the mad, a stigma based on the age-old belief that personal
sin caused insanity.[46] There also persisted the popular view of "the
asylum doctor as a sort of *petty sovereign*," who tyrannized his patients and his subordinates. This view, one doctor contended, was
extremely unfair and contrasted sharply with the real lot of an asy-

lum physician, which he described as a veritable *"via dolorosa"*; besides the physical violence and continual verbal threats, there were also the "anxieties and apprehensions" of administrative responsibilities.[47]

This latter domain was fraught with obstacles and frustrations. The public asylums were chronically underfunded. The government of Louis Philippe had ceded the financial initiative to build special hospitals for the insane to the *départements* in 1838. Yet one year later the same government cautioned the departmental prefects about the heavy expenditures required for construction and maintenance of these establishments, as if the parsimonious prefects had needed such reminders.[48] Consequently, as late as 1874 only forty of eighty-eight *départements* had special asylums for the insane, and hospital administrators found that the daily subsidy the prefect allocated for each patient was far too low to keep up with rising prices, compelling them to lower rations of food and wine.[49]

Psychiatrists objected to the central government leaving the public asylum system to function haltingly.[50] The initiative for reform, like that for financing, was left to the departmental prefects, with whom alienists had difficulty negotiating when improvements had to be made.[51] Worse, a decree by the new imperial government of Louis Napoleon on 25 March 1852 authorized the prefects to appoint asylum doctors. Brierre de Boismont believed that this decree would make physicians who owed their positions and their salaries to the prefects much more timid in requesting funding for improvements to their asylums.[52] The solution was patent, according to psychiatrists: the minister of interior ought to centralize the entire process of appointments, nominations, promotions, pensions, and salaries in order to assure the future of the asylum and its functionaries.[53]

Yet the most serious challenge psychiatry encountered was the rivalry presented by the clerical orders of the Catholic Church for most of the nineteenth century. After 1815 there was "a massive . . . expansion of religious facilities for the insane" coinciding with the emergence of psychiatry as a medical specialty. The nursing orders in particular thrived during the Restoration, "continued to hold their own under the July Monarchy, and . . . experienced a euphoric expansion" after the demise of the Second Republic. Priests, too, were inconveniences for physicians, posing a threat to medical authority in asylums. Friction between mental medicine and the Church, whose asylums abounded in provincial France, did not end with the 1838 law. Departmental prefects found clerically run mental hospitals to be relatively inexpensive and in some instances more congruent than secular hospitals with the Catholicism of the local population. "The flourishing" of clerical asylums in the 1840s indicates that the dispute between psychiatry and the clergy "was still fundamentally undecided."[54]

If their professional activities were hindered by a host of obstacles, alienists were no luckier in their relations with the rest of French medicine. Until 1877 there was no chair in mental pathology at the Paris faculty of medicine. There had been a chair from 1819 to 1822, but after student disturbances at the faculty in 1822 prompted Louis XVIII to suppress the teaching of medicine for a year, the chair in mental pathology was not renewed. For over fifty years lectures on psychological medicine formed no part of the official medical school curriculum and had to be delivered in asylums or in informal meetings. Most psychiatrists were first exposed to mental illness only after deciding to take up psychiatry as a career; that decision was possibly inspired by reading one of the classic texts on insanity by Pinel, Esquirol, Jean-Pierre Falret, Etienne Georget, or Louis Marcé. In the estimation of alienists other physicians were embarrassingly ignorant of madness. One psychiatrist echoed these impressions in 1876 when he wrote that "today, clinics in mental medicine are closed; medical students know nothing of the serious situations that engender insanity; and, tomorrow, when they confront the difficulties that await them, they will not be able to resolve them."[55]

To compound these problems, psychiatrists faced opposition to clinical teaching in the hospitals. The eminent Parisian alienist J. P. Falret (1794–1870) noted that in 1849 "in every country the authorities in general and many estimable doctors have protested against clinical lectures in mental medicine conducted inside asylums." It was alleged, Falret reported, that making the patient the object of public examination and introducing strangers (the students attending the lectures) into the hospitals would aggravate the illness. Falret dismissed these objections as groundless, but they were another source of embarrassment for the psychiatric profession, which saw clinical teaching as a symbol of its medical status and progress.[56]

Nineteenth-century French psychiatry prided itself on constituting a distinct branch of medicine but at the same time tried to foster closer ties to the rest of the medical profession. Calls for closer ties proliferated at midcentury. For example, J. P. Falret's son Jules (1824–1902), commenting on the relation between mental diseases and other affections of the nervous system, said that psychiatry's goal ought to be a firm union between "mental and general medicine,"[57] and Morel wrote that one of his chief aims was to link psychiatry more closely to general medicine than it had been before.[58]

French psychiatrists feared that their specialty was not considered a legitimate branch of medicine nor a legitimate biomedical science. These fears were undoubtedly justified to a large degree. Alienists themselves were unhappy with their reputation and viewed it as an obstacle to the attainment of the high medical status they believed their profession deserved.

Psychiatric Knowledge in the Nineteenth Century

The professional circumstances of alienism in the mid-1800s made it difficult for psychiatrists to depict themselves as genuine physicians. This difficulty increased when they were forced to conclude that they knew little about the somatic pathology and causes of a substantial number of abnormal affective states. The shifting trends of mainstream French medicine had cast doubt on psychiatry's claim that insanity was a physical disease like all others. As long as psychiatrists failed to substantiate this claim, their medical credentials were also in doubt, for they could not disprove the popular belief that madness was a spiritual or purely psychological condition. This failure meant that clerics were still entitled to diagnose and treat the insane.

The century had begun well for psychiatry. The fledgling specialty had been buoyed by the discovery in 1819 and 1822 of localized anatomical lesions in the brain membranes of the paralytic insane by two young Parisian doctors, Antoine-Laurent Bayle (1799–1858) and Louis Calmeil (1798–1859). In the 1820s and 1830s there was great enthusiasm among doctors who believed that further pathoanatomical research was all that was needed to discover the brain lesions of other psychological disturbances, such as melancholy, mania, and dementia. Their faith was consistent with the emphasis of the Paris school of clinical medicine on studying changes in diseased organic matter.[59] However, by the mid-1830s the passion for postmortem examinations of the sick had begun to decline. Many physicians believed that the study of pathological anatomy had unjustly overshadowed the study of insanity's causes and effective therapies.[60]

Psychiatrists of the same era agreed. That psychiatrists had shared the passion for pathological anatomy in the first place, despite the warnings of an authority like Pinel about its ultimately unedifying contributions to the study of insanity, is an indication of psychiatry's susceptibility to the trends in general medicine.[61] In any case, in the thirties and forties alienists duly took note of pathological anatomy's failure to find the structural lesions of the brain hoped for in earlier days. Perhaps the most influential voice was J. E. D. Esquirol's, Pinel's most famous psychiatric student and the unofficial leader of French alienists in the years after the fall of Napoleon I. In his *Mental Maladies* (1838), published two years before his death, Esquirol described the case of a maniac killed by a companion. The patient's body showed no lesions of the brain or of the cerebral membranes in autopsy. Esquirol wrote that

pathological anatomy, in spite of the very important labors of MM. Foville, Calmeil, Bayle, Guislain, etc. has not been able to make us acquainted with the organic cause of mania. Thirty years ago, I would willingly have written upon the pathological cause of madness. At the present day I would not attempt a labor so difficult—so much of incertitude and contradiction is there in the results of the necroscopy of the insane made up to this time.

Esquirol added that there was still reason to "hope for ideas more positive, more clear and more satisfactory." Yet his admission that he could no longer discuss the "pathological cause of madness" with the same confidence that he had before is evidence of psychiatry's uncertainty in the early 1840s.[62]

Other alienists criticised the pathoanatomical approach, including Ulysée Trélat (1795–1879)[63] and Brierre de Boismont, the latter of whom stated that he had "no reason to anticipate any satisfactory result from postmortem examinations of the insane with regard to hallucination; on this point we agree with the majority of the Faculty [of medicine]."[64] The attack on pathological anatomy in Parisian medicine coincided with the gradual decline in phrenology and in cerebral localization, the system of Franz Gall (1758–1828) and

Gaspar Spurzheim (1776–1832), who held that the different faculties of the mind could be localized in specific regions of the brain.

Phrenology never won the approval of the French scientific establishment,[65] but it had gained the support of the medical maverick François Broussais (1772–1838) in 1830 and was very popular among alienists of the period, including Esquirol, Etienne Georget (1795–1825), Brierre de Boismont, Guillaume Ferrus, and J. P. Falret. Some forty years later Falret remembered phrenology, like pathological anatomy, as a "general tendency" in mental medicine. Alienists looked to pathological anatomy to find the "primary reason for the phenomena observed in the mentally ill" and to phrenology to confirm that the material seat of insanity was in the brain. Gall's theory convinced many alienists that madness was caused by a physical injury to the brain.[66] The medical conviction that pathological anatomy would reveal the somatic origin in the brain of all types of mental disease and that phrenology proved that all psychical phenomena were localized in some region of the organ of thought tied psychiatrists to the major trend in early nineteenth-century Paris medicine and assured them of a biological context to account for the behavioral and affective phenomena of insanity.

The decline of phrenology and the Paris school of medicine, although hastened by certain psychiatrists, spelled trouble for alienism in general. A new theory of brain function that emerged with neurophysiologist Pierre Flourens (1794–1867) as its chief proponent scrutinized the sensory-motor functions of the nervous system, but not those of the organ of the mind. The hemispheres of the brain were viewed as the seat of perception, will, and intellect, but Flourens refused to consider any physiological connection between the senses and the brain itself, making it difficult for physicians to argue that mental functions could be tied to localized changes in brain structure and encouraging belief in the indivisibility of the mind and the unity of the soul.[67] Flourens's Cartesian dualism and his essentially theological brand of neurophysiology enjoyed the support of the French scientific establishment during the 1830s and 1840s.

The decline of phrenology, and the erosion of confidence in pathological anatomy made it more pressing for French psychiatry to face the problems that stemmed from the nature of psychiatric knowledge itself. What in fact was insanity, the disease asylum physicians were entrusted with curing? How did it differ from and how was it similar to the other diseases afflicting human beings? What were its symptoms? How were the different kinds of mental diseases differentiated and classified? What were their causes? Alienists' answers to these questions revealed how inexact the study of insanity was.

Psychiatrists, French or otherwise, insisted that insanity was a legitimate disease of the brain. As the authors of the 1874 report to the French minister of the interior on the national asylum system asserted, insanity developed under specific circumstances, like all other diseases, such as typhus in the army and gout in people with poor diets.[68] Louis Marcé (1828–1864) also emphasized the significance of viewing insanity as a disease. He wrote in 1862 that even "if the symptomatic elements [of madness] are less material" than those of other diseases, mental disorder "is nevertheless as easy to distinguish as fever."[69] The medical journalist Louis Peisse (1803–1880) noted too that many French alienists referred exclusively to the brain to account for the disturbances in instinct, passion, sentiment, and morality exhibited by the insane. Despite the indisputable role in mental illness of the organs of nutrition and reproduction as well as of the nervous system outside the brain and spinal cord, Peisse complained, psychiatrists were too "imbued" with the ideas of Gall and Georget and seemed preoccupied with restricting the physiology of mental phenomena to one organ.[70]

Unfortunately for psychiatrists, their belief in the cerebral origin of madness flew in the face of contemporaneous acknowledgement that the physiology of the brain and the manner in which it produced thought were still mysterious. If insanity were indeed a disease like all the others, its pathology had to be based on a physiological understanding of the brain, and even alienists had to acknowledge that for "all organs of the body except the brain great advances have been made in the knowledge of their physiological laws."[71] John Bucknill and Daniel Tuke claimed that while the understanding of the pathology of heart disease had progressed,

it is quite otherwise with the noble organ which lords it over the rest of the body. The mass of that which we call nerve-substance, because nerve-function is found to inhere thereto, possesses no adaptation which we can trace to the ends to which the Creator had made it subservient. An agglomeration of delicate cells in intimate connection with minute tubes or filaments, which communicate impressions made upon the cells at one end, to those cells which lie at their other extremities; this is the nervous apparatus. Its *modus operandi* is, and probably always will be, utterly unknown to us.[72]

Bucknill's and Tuke's French colleagues expressed similar sentiments. In 1856 Louis Delasiauve (1804–1893) argued that the mental operations in hallucinations could only be explained on the basis of the interaction of body and mind. Yet, Delasiauve declared, this interaction was far from clear.[73] There was no scientifically satisfactory explanation that could bridge the gap between the physiology of the brain and the psychological phenomena that even the most skeptical of doctors attributed to that organ.

Given this lack of satisfactory explanation, alienists could not plausibly reduce mental symptoms to either the pathological anatomy or pathophysiology of the brain. Nor is there any reason to believe they wished to do so even if somatic pathology were clearer, for it would have meant reducing insanity's symptoms to epiphenomenal status. As the German alienist Wilhelm Griesinger (1817–1868)[74] wrote in 1861, only a "flat and shallow materialism" endeavors to derive "the endless variety of thoughts, feelings, and desires, not only of individual men, but of different ages" from "the elementary phenomena which occur in the nerve-masses." He, too, could think of insanity as nothing else than "an affection of the brain." However, he realized that cerebral pathology

is, even in the present day, to a great extent in the same state which the pathology of the thoracic organs was in before the days of [René] Laennec. Instead of proceeding in every case from the changes of structure of the organ, and being able to deduce in an exact manner the production of the symptoms from the changes in the tissue, it has very often to deal with symptoms of which it can scarcely give an approximation to the seat, and of whose mode of origin it is totally ignorant. It must keep to the external phenomena, and establish the groups of diseases according to something common and characteristic in the symptoms altogether independently of their anatomical basis.[75]

Griesinger's comments echoed those of his French colleagues. Although he called himself a "somaticist," he, like J. P. Falret, believed that the psychological irregularities and mood disorders characterizing madness were the most important clinical phenomena for psychiatrists.[76] According to Jules Falret, Griesinger was to be applauded for pointing out that "psychical phenomena" constituted a highly important part of the study of lunacy "without which our specialty would cease to exist as a distinct science and would come to be incorporated entirely into cerebral pathology."[77] Indeed, Griesinger had argued in 1861 that psychiatry "must assert the position so lately obtained for it," and "any attempt to obliterate" the difference between it and cerebral pathology would undermine this achievement.[78]

The nineteenth-century French psychiatrist confronted a dilemma: as a physician he was compelled to consider the somatic mechanisms underlying mental disorders, although these processes remained obscure; yet for psychiatry to be a distinct branch of medicine it was necessary to emphasize the psychological symptoms of madness such as hallucinations, illusions, depression, and disturbances of memory, judgment, and comprehension. But recourse to morbid psychology as the appropriate context for psychiatry proved to be no more satisfactory than recourse to pathological anatomy or pathophysiology. By devoting such a significant part of his specialty to the study of behavioral and affective phenomena the alienist either tacitly or explicitly permitted philosophical considerations to influence his diagnosis of insanity. For example, Bucknill and Tuke admitted that a psychiatrist "must not only be a physician, but a metaphysician."[79] Brierre de Boismont agreed for the most part. He argued that

to us, as to millions, man is an intelligence served by organs; to account only for the latter, would be to tear a quill from the pinion of spiritual activity. If there be one branch of medicine in which this opinion would offer the strangest paradox, without doubt it is that of mental diseases. They incessantly oblige the physician to resort to the most difficult metaphysical problems. . . .

We therefore consider ourselves following out the truth, in maintaining the necessity of allying philosophy and medicine, especially in mental maladies . . .[80]

Although Brierre de Boismont would have disagreed with Bucknill's and Tuke's solutions to the "metaphysical problems" of psychological medicine, they all agreed that it was nearly impossible to eliminate philosophic considerations from the study of madness as long as its symptoms consisted of derangements of reason and acts of questionable morality.

Given this feature of insanity's symptomatology, it was doubtless just as hard to distinguish reason from madness. Throughout most of the nineteenth century, French doctors conceded that there was no definitive line of demarcation between the two mental states.[81] Emile Renaudin (1808–1865) explained that the analogies between mental alienation and sanity were so striking that only the trained eye of the experienced clinician could distinguish between normal and deviant mental states.[82] Yet in appealing solely to the experience of the alienist in the diagnosis of madness, Renaudin fell far short of providing a convincing standard according to which, for example, a hallucination could be judged to be pathological.

Another point of psychiatric imprecision was the classification of the varieties of insanity. Most physicians at midcentury acknowledged that a nosology of lunacy based on organic lesions was impractical; yet at the same time it was felt that the classification systems of Pinel and Esquirol were outdated. This confusion and the resulting conflict were evident during the psychiatric debates over the classification of mental diseases in the 1860s. Some blamed the disagreements among alienists on the nature of insanity itself. Delasiauve admitted that in psychological medicine an organization of the clinical facts into neatly defined categories was not possible. He preferred the retention of the standard classification system, in which monomania, melancholy, mania, dementia, and imbecility or idiocy were distinct groups, because in the absence of firm knowledge of their causes, these categories at least had the advantage of being founded on readily distinguishable clusters of symptoms.[83] Unfortunately, as his critics pointed out, the succession and variability of symptoms over time hardly conformed to the standard method of classification. The same mentally ill patient often exhibited such a wide range of symptoms during hospitalization that only an arbitrary decision could define him or her as manic or melancholic. This clinical phenomenon had puzzled B. A. Morel early in his career and prompted him to conclude that mania and melancholy were symptoms of one nervous affection rather than two fixed and distinct nosological classes.[84]

Jules Falret argued that the customary method of classifying the varieties of insanity justified Morel's criticism that doctors were not aware of the entire sequence of symptoms in each patient's illness. The result, Falret charged, was that the asylum psychiatrist confines himself most often to noting the mental state in which a patient finds himself at the moment of his entry into the asylum, without worrying if this state will undergo transformations, and without studying the different phases through which this same patient passes in the subsequent years of his illness. If he leaves the asylum and returns there later in a different mental state [the alienist] confines himself almost always to determining this new state, without relating it to that which the same patient presented previously. In a word, the present is rarely associated with the past or future in the study of mental maladies.

Falret concluded that this "psychological doctrine" presented "serious inconveniences" in the observation and the classification of mental diseases.[85]

The alienist J. B. Parchappe recognized also that there was little consensus among psychiatrists on the nature of mental alienation. He attributed this lack to the state of biomedical science and noted that psychiatrists needed a general concept to impose scientific unity on the myriad organic and psychological characteristics and on the pathological development of insanity. Without one, according to Parchappe, "divergences" of opinion among doctors would continue, further postponing the development of a viable classification of mental illnesses.[86]

Morel's advocacy of a new classification of mental diseases based on causes was a promising innovation for midcentury psychiatrists. When alienists wrote about causality, they ordinarily drew up long lists of causes embracing a wide range of factors. The French seemed to be particularly prone to this exercise. Griesinger maintained that French alienists were guilty of erecting "abstract tables of physical and moral* causes" and hence did not explore the pathogeny and etiology of insanity as deeply as the Germans.[87] Despite drawing Baillarger's objections, Griesinger seems to have been correct. The cataloguing of causes proved to be susceptible to abuse, as the alienist Jacques Moreau de Tours (1804–1884) pointed out in 1845:

---

*The term *moral* employed by Pinel and his successors in psychiatry is not strictly equivalent to the modern term *psychological;* alienists used it to denote the passions and emotions rather than the psychological faculties such as memory, imagination, reason, attention, or judgment. See Kathleen M. Grange, "Pinel and Eighteenth-Century Psychiatry," *Bulletin of the History of Medicine* 35 (1961):442–53.

There is no lack of causes of mental illness collected by authors. But these cases, although eloquent on many points, are mute on others. Each observer has accepted them from his particular point of view. He only has seen the aspects in line with his theories; the other facts have completely escaped him or remained in half obscurity, impenetrable and sterile. He has described them as he has seen them, incompletely. The imprint of his convictions is evident in each line. Compare the observations that have been conveyed to us by the partisans of the predominance of mental etiology regarding the dynamic or functional nature of mental change with those observations of the supporters of physical causes, of the organic nature of intellectual lesions; everything that supports the dominant idea is related precisely and in detail; the remainder is hardly indicated or not at all.[88]

There was much truth to Moreau's observation. In many instances it appeared that the cataloguing of insanity's causes was a neoscholastic exercise involving little more than equivocation over words. There were also inherent difficulties in drawing clearly the pathogeny of mental alienation: the specification of each cause and its relative influence was so inexact an enterprise that an alienist was virtually free to indulge his own tastes and preconceived ideas.

Finally, there lurked the possibility that physicians might be tempted to take the unjustified step of equating the cause of insanity with its essential nature. For instance, Baillarger claimed that there were some who confused the notion of cause with the somatic condition of madness.[89] There were precedents in medicine for confusion of this sort; Parchappe recalled, for example, that "the humoral theory of antiquity" had led many to believe that the causes of disease were the humors themselves. This, Parchappe stressed, was sloppy thinking, and he warned against medical acceptance of Morel's etiological method of classifying mental diseases.[90]

Nevertheless, some psychiatrists agreed with Morel that beyond the unedifying litany of physical and psychological causes conventionally cited by alienists there had to be a fundamental, unitary, and "imperishable" lesion that explained both the etiology and the nature of mental illness. Charles Lasègue (1816–1883), who later would be named chief physician for the insane at the Paris prefecture of police, saw Moreau's research as an attempt to realize the "pathologist's dream," as he called it, of reducing all the chaotic symptoms and conditions of insanity to one prototypical lesion.[91]

The overall picture of nineteenth-century French psychiatric

ideas that emerges is one of uncertainty, imprecision, and disagreement. While many alienists were attracted to Morel's advice
that they base the classification of mental diseases on etiological
principles, others, like Delasiauve, remained wedded to the no-
sologies of Pinel and Esquirol. Physicians did seem to agree that
insanity was a certifiable disease with its seat in the brain, but this
conviction was hard to sustain in the face of the anatomical and
pathophysiological evidence of the time. It simply could not be
verified that madness was as much a disease of the body as was
pneumonia or chronic fever with their characteristic and distinguishable somatic lesions, nor were the findings of biomedical science consistent enough to justify drawing firm connections between emotional disorders and organic lesions—there were only
educated guesses about how the brain functioned in abnormal mental states.

It is significant, then, that psychiatrists were noticeably concerned with proving insanity's somatic nature, although in the era
before germ theory many other diseases were defined according to
external symptoms and not according to organic physiological
causes.[92] This tendency to believe in a somatic theory of insanity
did not escape the attention of contemporaries like Peisse[93] or the
doctor who denounced the inadequacies of pathological anatomy
and the way in which psychiatrists nonetheless placed so much
stock in it:

Alienists seem to believe that they would see more clearly [in their
pathoanatomical research] if cerebral functions were less delicate; I am
sorry to deprive them of this consolation, but I shall supply them with
another: pathological anatomy casts no more light on the diseases of other
organs. . . . [A]natomical lesions ordinarily maintain no relationship to
functional lesions that is detectable by our senses.[94]

It can only be concluded that psychiatrists continued to feel that
the identification of a physical cause of madness was crucial to their
specialty. Without it psychiatrists stood to lose professional advantages. Because psychological states constituted the primary clinical
focus of psychiatry, there was always the threat that nonmedical
people could justify their intervention in the diagnosis of insanity
unless physicians could show that its causes were ultimately organic
in nature. Thus the alienist Griesinger felt compelled to deride
purely psychological approaches to insanity; to his mind, they over-

looked "the organic causes" of lunacy, "looking only to the intellectual side, regarding them as the results of former moral conflicts."[95]
Griesinger's comments suggest the dilemma in which midcentury
psychiatrists found themselves: the only way to ward off nonmedical
involvement in the diagnosis of insanity was to claim for the disease
a somatic pathology that remained highly problematic.

The same was true for nonmedical intervention in the treatment
and management of madness. Without proof that insanity was due
to somatic causes, there was no reason why physicians should enjoy exclusive rights to cure and care for the insane. The result was
a pervasive doubt at midcentury that certain mental states constituted legitimate objects for medical scrutiny and that deviant
mental function could be explained in terms of brain anatomy and
physiology.[96] As long as this doubt existed, psychiatry's putative
hegemony over the diagnosis and treatment of insanity would be
vulnerable to criticism and challenges from lay and clerical communities.

The Founding of the Annales
médico-psychologiques

The turmoil and cognitive disorientation in psychiatry in the 1840s
and 1850s reflected the changes French medicine in general was
undergoing at the same time. Dissatisfaction with the Ventôse law,
the continuing existence of the *officiers de santé*, and the growing
wave of quackery and charlatanism reached a peak in these years. In
addition, overcrowding within the profession fostered a stubborn
individualism among physicians and created a highly competitive
atmosphere and substantial economic inequalities. It may not be an
exaggeration to describe the 1840s as a decade of crisis for French
medicine.[97] The 1840s were "decisive years" for teachers, lawyers,
civil servants, writers, and architects as well. "Like their counter-
parts in England and the United States," professionals in France
spent the decade trying to form organizations that defined and restricted access to occupational groups. French physicians specifically sought to foster "the spirit of association" within their ranks in
order to quell the disagreements that hamstrung their efforts to
establish their social status on the basis of a commonly accepted
body of expert knowledge.[98]

During this unstable period, when medicine was undergoing "a crisis of identity," the first volume of the *Annales médico-psycholo-giques* appeared in January 1843. Before this date, mental patholo-gists had no specifically psychiatric journal in which to publish their work; the *Annales* provided a forum for alienists. The original edito-rial board consisted of Laurent Cerise, who edited the articles deal-ing with general medicopsychological topics; Jules Baillarger, who edited materials concerning mental alienation strictly speaking; and F. A. Longet (1811–1871), who edited works on the structure, func-tion, and pathology of the nervous system.

Cerise (1807–1869) was a physician deeply interested in nervous diseases, particularly in the relations between body and mind. He outlined the objectives and themes of the *Annales* in his introduc-tion to the first volume.[99] He paid homage to Pinel whose ideas, he wrote, more or less constituted the ethos of the new *Annales*. It was Pinel who had challenged the traditional theories of insanity and had urged that it be distinguished from crime and other forms of social deviance. However, Cerise continued, the time had passed since an exclusively alienist journal was warranted. "The science of mental alienation exists today without dispute," he triumphantly declared.[100] Never before had insanity been the object of so much medical study. The future was limitless for psychiatry. Great clini-cal discoveries remained to be made, and there was still progress to be made in the institutional care of the insane. Therefore, he stated, the new journal would be addressed not only to physicians but also to legislators and administrators, who had much to contribute to the understanding and treatment of madness. Cerise argued that be-cause mental alienation was closely tied to the anatomy, physiol-ogy, and pathology of the nervous system it formed a part of "the science of the relations between body and mind" and was bound to attract the attention of many nonalienists—such as Cerise himself.

Consequently, Cerise called for the intervention of philosophy in scientific research. He rejected metaphysics and psychological the-ories that ignored laws governing the operations of organized mat-ter.[101] But he also rejected the "school of ideologues" who depicted mental activity as only the product of bodily mechanisms. The mind-body issue was clouded in confusion, he admitted, and it served no constructive purpose to view it from only one perspec-tive. He referred to the conflict raging between the spiritualist and materialist schools as examples of this form of dogmatism. Spiritu-alists in early nineteenth-century France tended to regard the mind as ultimately independent of the body and the laws governing the physical world.[102] Only by examining men and women from the point of view of the "duality" of body and mind could progress be made, Cerise maintained.[103]

When he turned his attention to the question of mental alienation, Cerise noted the stalemate in psychiatric theory by the early 1840s. He applauded the endeavors of Pinel and his disciples to improve the custodial care of the insane but also lamented that they had not submitted the various forms of madness to "methodical observation." Testifying to the profound midcentury disagreements over the interpretation of insanity and its etiology, Cerise stressed that there was a great need for a "general doctrine of mental alienation" with which to order all the facts systematically. This was especially true in 1843, Cerise declared, because of the proliferation of different theories within mental medicine: the patho-anatomical school viewed lunacy as a structural and organic disease amenable only to physical therapy; the psychological school recommended "moral treatment" exclusively, on the grounds that insanity was a disease of the soul or pure mind; the vitalist school employed both physical and moral techniques but restricted themselves to moderating the symptoms rather than combatting the disease itself. Cerise reasoned that the only way to end this state of affairs was to resort to careful clinical observation. However, recognizing that the strict observation of insanity entailed numerous difficulties, he advised pathologists to use hypotheses in studying its symptoms. Anticipating the ideas of the physiologist Claude Bernard, a contributor to the second volume of the *Annales médico-psychologiques*,[104] Cerise wrote that hypotheses were crucial to the scientific observation and appreciation of phenomena, for without them there could be little order in the way the empirical data were gathered.[105] In order to achieve any future success, mental pathology had to be committed to the clinical accumulation and analysis of the phenomena according to a common observational method, commitment to which, he admitted ruefully, most doctors of his day were "hostile" or "unfaithful."[106]

Because the *Annales médico-psychologiques* was to be a journal devoted to the study of the relation between body and mind, Cerise announced, it would also necessarily touch on questions of legal medicine. He was not unaware of the possibilities of conflict between doctors and French magistrates, a tension that had characterized the involvement of psychiatrists in judicial proceedings for the previous twenty-five years. Jurists and the public disliked psychiatric use of the insanity defense because they suspected that physicians denied the existence of free will, but Cerise claimed he had no intention of undermining the notion of free will, one of "the doctrines without which society could not exist."[107] He simply expressed his hope that studies published in the *Annales* would help to clarify the problems surrounding the legal responsibility of criminals.

Cerise also saw the *Annales médico-psychologiques* as a means for shedding light on nervous diseases, among which he included hysteria, hypochondria, epilepsy, catalepsy, and somnambulism. Nervous diseases occupied a crucial position in the relationship between body and mind, he wrote. They shared many characteristics with mental alienation, such as hallucinations, and were in need of close observation by mental pathologists as much as mental diseases were. Cerise noted that although nervous affections had been the object of medical scrutiny longer than insanity, they were much less understood. Here, too, the various medical theories had done little to edify practitioners, with the result that all too often the question of nervous illnesses was left to nonphysicians. Cerise lamented that organized medicine preferred to ignore the elusive and hard-to-decipher phenomena of nervous ailments and thereby gave up an important opportunity to improve public health and to learn more about mind-body relations.[108]

Cerise's introduction is significant because it reflected the intellectual state of French medicine in general and alienism in particular in 1843. General ideas about pathology were changing, yet many physicians continued to side dogmatically with one medical faction or another. Like other French physicians, Cerise distrusted the organic theories of the physiologists Gall, Pierre Cabanis, Broussais, and Georget. He felt that the study of the organism ought not to be limited to the consideration of physical properties alone but should encompass all the phenomena of life, including the full range of mental activities, intellectual and affective. He hoped that in this way the operations of the mind would not be reduced to the functions of the brain, a "materialist error" he attributed to Gall. As he argued in 1842, the nervous system constituted the link between phenomena of a purely mental and physical nature. Its study, he wrote, demonstrated the influence of moral factors on physiological characteristics and hence the distinctive nature of human spiritual activity.[109] The physiologist, Cerise argued, interpreted all mental life as the result of physical causes originating either in the viscera or the encephalon,[110] yet there was no doubting that the organic composition of the brain that predisposed an individual to a particular way of thinking or feeling was also subject to a large extent to "the modifying authority" of "the moral and intellectual environment" of society. Cerise thus concluded that the moral conditions of public life exercised a great influence over mental health.[111]

As founder and editor of the new *Annales médico-psychologiques,* Cerise's ecletic position on the delicate mind-body issue for the most part represented the outlook of midcentury mental medicine. It was also a politically judicious position for the editor of a fledgling medical journal to take, for the issue of the mind's relation to the body was highly contentious in early nineteenth-century France. The issue had become heavily politicized by the 1840s, with many orthodox scholars and clerics complaining that because physicians subscribed to anticlerical and liberal ideas, they reduced the mind's functions to the operations of the brain.[112] Like many alienists, Cerise saw the pathoanatomical approach as outdated, but he did not overlook the importance of organic conditions in disease. For example, he conceded that in insanity it was the brain that was diseased and not the mind or soul, an important consideration for psychiatrists who saw the physical reality of madness as the primary justification for medical rather than religious intervention in the treatment of the insane.[113] His emphasis on the pathogenic influence of moral factors was also consistent with alienist etiological interpretations in 1843.[114] Yet Cerise rejected the purely psychological method of academic philosophy cultivated by Victor Cousin and his followers, which ignored the many points of contact between the mind and the body.[115] For Cerise, this approach was as dogmatic as the physiological theories popular a generation earlier. Cerise was careful to distance himself and the *Annales* from physiological ideas that had received official condemnation from political and academic quarters without denying the imperative of organized medicine to study and minister to the diseased body. He patently tried to transcend the metaphysical and political disputes by cultivating the image of a value-free approach to the mind-body issue that would not antagonize official opinion and thus jeopardize his new journal.

Cerise's flexible approach also mirrored the "eclecticism" of Paris medicine in its fourth and last stage of supremacy in the 1840s. Many French physicians were skeptical of the value of theories and instead were committed to medical research from a wide variety of experimental perspectives.[116] Cerise agreed that theories hitherto borrowed from general medicine had not succeeded in solving the riddle of madness and its treatment. His recommendation that psychiatrists consult the writings of nonalienists and seriously concern themselves with nervous disorders indicates that he and many psychiatrists believed that more study was warranted if physicians hoped to escape the intellectual impasse in which they found themselves in the 1840s.

The founding of the *Annales médico-psychologiques* was yet another indication that the mid-nineteenth century was a period of transition and unrest for French psychiatry. Many alienists were dissatisfied with the sectarianism and factionalism that had characterized the profession in the years between the Napoleonic regime and the early 1840s. Unsure of where psychiatry was headed in the future, they were nonetheless certain that things had to change dramatically. Discontented with the state of professional practice, alienists also saw themselves as assuming an almost impossible therapeutic responsibility within the asylum, a responsibility they sensed neither the public nor other doctors regarded highly. Equally disturbing was the awareness that their claims to positive knowledge of insanity rang hollow. As long as alienists could not make these claims convincingly, they had no rationale for exercising exclusive diagnostic and therapeutic jurisdiction over the insane. By the end of the century French psychological medicine was firmly established within a culture that placed credence in psychiatric explanations and freely borrowed medical or pathological metaphors to describe social and political phenomena. Yet that should not obscure the fact that most French psychiatrists were restless and unsure of the future at midcentury. It was the response of psychiatry to this troubled period that laid the groundwork for the relative acceptance of mental medicine by 1900.

Chapter Two

François Leuret and Medical
Opposition to
Moral Treatment, 1835–1850

The gaps in French psychiatric knowledge at midcentury left alienists vulnerable to clerical allegations that medicine did not deserve exclusive rights to the institutional treatment and care of the insane. Particularly upsetting to many psychiatrists was that the Catholic Church's belief that insanity warranted moral therapies appeared to be vindicated by some alienists, principally François Leuret (1797–1851). Largely because of Leuret's efforts in the 1830s and 1840s, there was renewed interest in moral treatment, an approach to madness that advocated primarily psychological methods of therapy such as reasoning, kindness, and persuasion. However, moral treatment also called into question the efficacy of conventional medical therapies such as drugs, setons, and bleeding. It therefore posed a challenge to psychological medicine, most of whose practitioners were keen on establishing that madness was a somatic disease that only physicians, not priests or nuns, were qualified to treat. Leuret's version of moral treatment denied the practical importance of the somatic theory of insanity and thus angered his fellow alienists, who criticized him for implying that the Church was entitled to treat the mentally ill.

François Leuret was born 30 December 1797, one of six children of a baker from Nancy. In 1816 he went to Paris to study medicine but shortly after his arrival discovered that his father refused to support his studies. Leuret instead joined the departmental army of the Meurthe, which was soon to be garrisoned at Saint-Dénis. Unsuited to military life, he attended daily courses at the Paris Faculty of Medicine, where he showed an aptitude for the study of the illnesses of the mind. He later secured an internship at Charenton hospital under the devoutly religious Antoine Royer-Collard (1768–1825), and in 1826 he defended his medical thesis. After a brief stay in Nancy, he returned to Paris in 1828 and assumed a post at Esquirol's *maison de santé*. Esquirol appointed Leuret the chief editor of the *Annales d'hygiène publique et de médecine légale,* the organ for the influential French public hygiene movement and the so-called Esquirol circle.[1] Leuret also directed another private asylum in Paris and became a ward head at Bicêtre.[2]

Leuret's early reverses in life left him a proud, impatient, and independent man. His fierce devotion to work, by all accounts, contributed to the decline of his health after 1848 and to his premature death in 1851. His good friend Ulysée Trélat recalled that Leuret's daily walks into Paris and back to his barracks at Saint-Dénis were long and arduous; even as a young man Leuret suffered from heart palpitations and breathlessness. As a practicing psychiatrist with a growing clientele, Leuret's daily routine got no easier. His day began at six; after spending the morning at Bicêtre, he would go to his private *maison de santé* to treat patients until evening; at home he would devote the evening to study and writing. In addition to articles and editorial work for the *Annales d'hygiène publique et de médecine légale,* he published antiphrenological tracts and a two-volume work on the comparative anatomy of the nervous system. But it was his two books on the psychology and treatment of insanity that caused the most commotion.

The first of these was his *Psychological Fragments on Insanity* of 1834.[3] According to Alexandre Brierre de Boismont, this was Leuret's first important work on mental alienation, one that anticipated much of his later theory of moral treatment.[4] In it Leuret argued that insanity was only the exaggeration of an error in thinking and that the normal operations of the mind were the most appropriate standard by which to judge the pathological extent of a hallucinatory delusion.[5] For Trélat, Leuret's book was important because

after the abuse in science of reducing everything, so to speak, to the appreciation of material phenomena, this volume forced the issue and enlarged the field of study. Instead of making the disease [of insanity] something completely exceptional, François Leuret, the author, insisted on viewing it as a modification of health in which are found in most cases tendencies, particular forms, exaggeration, and the most delicate nuances of the normal state [of psychological functioning].[6]

Leuret did not deny that mental derangement was tied to organic changes in the brain. However, he believed that since the cause of insanity was unknown, it was best not to persist in characterizing madness as a somatic condition.[7]

The therapeutic implications of this viewpoint became clear in his *Moral Treatment* (1840). There he argued that insanity, as an "aberration of the faculties of understanding," was not "like ordinary diseases, characterized by physical symptoms; and the causes that produce it, when from time to time appreciable to the senses, belong most often to an order of phenomena completely foreign to the general laws of matter: these are the passions and ideas." Again Leuret stated that ideas, passions, or the mental faculties never manifested themselves without the intervention of the nervous system.[8] For purposes of treatment this truth was of little significance, for it did not necessarily prove that an "organic brain lesion" was the immediate cause of lunacy.[9] Because psychological and emotional states constituted the most obvious and numerous symptoms of madness, it seemed far more logical to Leuret to employ all the methods that "act directly on the intelligence and the passions," rather than the bleeding, purgatives, diuretics, and pharmaceutical preparations customarily used by most physicians.[10]

Leuret was not content simply to criticize the physicalist medical therapy that he felt dominated the curative endeavors of his alienist colleagues. He also directed his attacks against specific physicians. He chastised J. P. Falret for failing to make good his promise of 1822 to prove through pathological anatomy that a lesion of the encephalon occurred in every emotional disorder.[11] He derided phrenologically oriented psychiatrists, such as Guillaume Ferrus, Jean Baptiste Parchappe, and Jacques Etienne Belhomme, for their insistence that madness could be anatomically localized in specific regions of the brain.[12] But he directed his real ire at what he called the Charenton school, physicians such as Jacques Moreau de Tours, Louis Calmeil, and Antoine-Laurent Bayle,[13] and the Salpêtrière school, physicians such as Falret, Etienne Georget (1795–1828),

Achille Foville (1799–1878),* and Félix Voisin.[14] Leuret accused
these doctors of subordinating Pinel's moral treatment to physicalist remedies, a practice also deplored in 1840 by a physician, who
had worked under Leuret at Bicêtre.[15] Their prejudices, Leuret
alleged, were based on the conviction that a pathological alteration
of the brain preceded every morbid operation of the mind and that
therefore the target for the alienist physician ought to be the organic processes of the "animal economy."[16] Leuret saw this orientation as a grave error because it reinforced the view that the insane
were incurable.[17] It also prompted the kind of question posed by
Leuret's admirer Louis Delasiauve in 1860: if madness was little
more than the result of "congestive inflammation" of the brain,
why were cures so rare and transitory when anti-inflammatory
treatment was applied?[18]

By all accounts, Leuret's criticisms of the frequency of physicalist
therapy in French mental hospitals were justified. Pinel had introduced a moral treatment in the 1790s at Bicêtre and Salpêtrière
and recommended its radical use in cases of insanity without paralysis and dementia because he detested the physical brutality and was
suspicious of the medical therapies used to treat the insane in most
eighteenth-century asylums.[19] Yet despite the many acknowledg-
ments of Pinel's benevolence and innovative improvements in psychiatric care, many of his successors were skeptical that moral treatment was as effective as Pinel claimed. Their skepticism may have
been a reaction to the conclusions Pinel drew from his success with
moral treatment; he wrote in his *Treatise on Insanity* (1801) that
"the successful application of moral regimen exclusively, gives great
weight to the supposition, that, in a majority of instances, there is
no organic lesion of the brain nor of the cranium."[20] This conclusion's implicit challenge to prevailing medical theory was reinforced by Pinel's admission of moral treatment's "non-esoteric, lay
origins."[21] In the face of such statements, even as admiring a follower as Esquirol did not dispense with pharmaceutical and other
physicalist remedies. Similarly, in 1820 Etienne Georget, a pivotal
figure in early nineteenth-century alienism, declared his support
for treatment directed toward eliminating the lesion of the diseased
organ. Like Esquirol, Georget praised moral methods such as isola-

---

*Not to be confused with his son, also named Achille (1831–1887).

tion within a medically supervised institution but also clung to his belief in remedies applied to the body.[22] Georget seemed to be wary of exclusive use of moral treatment because it suggested that he was no longer concerned with the somatic condition of his patient. Thus, if a form of moral treatment was practiced in French asylums in Leuret's day, it was, as Parchappe explained, an impersonal and collective therapy based on the patient's compliance with hospital regulations and obedience to the administrative authority of the asylum doctor.[23] Psychiatrists, faced with mounting numbers of hospitalized patients, abandoned individualistic care and equated moral treatment solely with the surveillance and management of large groups of patients. It was also often eclipsed by the traditional therapies central to the alienist's therapeutic arsenal throughout the nineteenth century.[24] Ludger Lunier explained, for example, that the "sequestration" of the insane in hospitals as an exclusive means of therapy implied the renunciation of the rules guiding the treatment of other diseases.[25] Asylum doctors did not want to practice moral treatment alone for fear of losing their medical image as ministers to the body of the madman.

Leuret seemed to take a perverse satisfaction in relating the opposition his ideas met within medical circles. He noted that his moral treatment—especially intimidation or "moral revulsion" through the liberal use of cold showers—was resisted by other physicians and that his views were labeled at the Royal Academy of Medicine as retrograde, dangerous, harking back to the days before Pinel, when the insane were chained and locked up in dark cells.[26] Leuret also quoted Louis Calmeil, who accused him of depicting the mind as an "independent principle, situated outside the influence of the brain." According to Leuret, Calmeil believed that a doctor was obliged to take into account all the physical changes and "dispositions" of the body and that through the treatment of these elements the alienist could best undermine "the infirmities of reason."[27] Leuret's own impression was that the discussion of his ideas was far from objective and disinterested.[28]

Was Leuret's perception of the situation accurate? Was the reaction of the medical establishment as pronounced and negative as he characterized it? Leuret's innovations did send reverberations throughout the Paris medical community, for in their eulogies to Leuret in 1851 both Brierre de Boismont and Trélat testified that Leuret had been the target of unaccustomed criticism from his colleagues.[29] Emile Renaudin also wrote that the debate over moral therapy was not always conducted according to strictly empirical and scientific considerations.[30] Leuret prompted a particularly splenetic response from the private asylum doctor Esprit Blanche, who had delivered a paper to the Academy of Medicine in 1839 in answer to Leuret's two papers in 1838 that detailed several supposed cures with moral treatment.[31] According to the academy's report, Leuret's papers created a considerable stir because at least one of the cases Leuret mentioned involved such prolonged harassment of the patient and such marked swings between kindness and overt mental cruelty that Blanche likened it to the treatment of the mad in pre-Pinel hospitals. Blanche feared that such an approach would become a general doctrine among alienists.[32] His apprehensions were shared by Dr. Pariset and Dr. Esquirol, who filed the report on Blanche's paper at the academy. Pariset condemned Leuret's reliance on intimidation and summarized what he deemed the proper treatment of the insane:

There are . . . two things that ought never to be lost sight of; I mean, a precept and a maxim. The precept is to favor the renewal of the organs by keeping all the excretionary pores open and introducing into the [animal] economy the materials appropriate for [organic] composition. . . . The maxim is to make yourself the sole authority for your patients in a way that is dignified for them and for you; the sole authority to whom they surrender themselves, for this surrender of their being is the result of their confidence and the respect that one inspires in them. Yet you will only secure this authority, confidence, and respect through justice and kindness. . . . It is through these rewards alone that their hearts will be open to you, that their reason will be docile to your advice and will submit to yours; whereas to adopt a code of conduct dominated by harshness towards them is to prepare oneself for the cruelest disappointments. Misunderstood by your assistants and students, this harshness soon degenerates into barbarism.[33]

Pariset, like many of his colleagues in organized medicine, believed that the best interests of the insane lay in the trained physician's use of somatic remedies, such as drugs and bleeding, and his complete authority over his patients in a hospital setting. Only in this way, most physicians were convinced, would the insane receive genuinely benevolent and effective care.

The discussion that followed the report on Blanche's paper revealed little more sympathy for Leuret than that found in Pariset's report. One doctor approved wholeheartedly of the medical advice to stimulate excretions with drugs, "one of the most powerful means of cure;" another declared that "almost all doctors engaged in the treatment of madness" used purgatives to some extent.[34] The message was clear: many doctors disapproved of Leuret's apparent lack of benevolence toward the insane and his reluctance to employ therapeutic measures directly affecting the body.

However, Leuret was not one to let the matter rest there. On 2 February 1841 he delivered a paper to the academy and entitled it "Moral Revulsion in the Treatment of Insanity." As Dr. François Double noted, the paper had attracted "sustained attention" and "lively and prolonged interest," underlining the importance of Leuret's ideas to French medicine.[35] Double cited Leuret's contention that moral treatment should not be employed when a physical cause clearly determined the onset of delirium because in these cases moral means were largely useless compared to somatic medical therapy. Double saw this as proof that Leuret was not dogmatic about the treatment of insanity. After all, Double went on, to hold that only moral therapy was sufficient to treat madness would constitute a "veritable fraud," for

by an inevitable consequence of this principle the insane would lay no claim to any pharmaceutical care [and] the study and treatment of every alteration of the intellectual faculties would soon escape the domain of medicine; philosophers, moralists, and theologians would hasten to assume the prerogatives [of treatment and diagnosis]. Science and humanity would suffer equally.

There were other good reasons for not adopting moral treatment exclusively, Double added. The history of medicine had many examples of madness that seemed to be both caused and cured by physical conditions: there were women who became disturbed each time they were pregnant and who were cured only after delivery; there was Richard Mead's case of a maniacal woman cured of her mental derangement when she contracted abdominal dropsy. Similarly, Peruvian bark had proven to be effective in tempering the intermittent crises of partial insanity. Who could deny, Double asked, that monomania, "which seems to belong most closely to the moral domain," was often accompanied by disturbances in organic function, such as insomnia, constipation, and diarrhea? Just as the mind exercised an incontestable influence over the body, Double reasoned, so it was pure folly for doctors to ignore the therapeutic implications of the influence of the body on the mind.[36]

Despite the judicious treatment Leuret received from Double, certain doctors at the academy refused to acknowledge his distinction between psychical disorders with and without somatic lesions, and hence his distinction between cases in which moral or medical therapies ought to be applied. His most vocal critic was Guillaume Ferrus. A former student of Pinel, Ferrus was, with the death of Esquirol in 1840, arguably the most important psychiatrist in France. In 1835 he had been named inspector-general of insane asylums in France and was a major consultant in the drafting of the 1838 law regarding the national system of public assistance to the insane. He founded the innovative Sainte-Anne farm, where he experimented with work therapy for the mad. He was also one of the founding members of the Société médico-psychologique and presided at its first meeting on 26 April 1852. Ferrus believed that Leuret's opinions were "erroneous in principle and in practice."[37] He claimed that Leuret was vague about when moral treatment was to be superseded by medical therapy or when both were to be used jointly. In any case, Ferrus continued, Leuret was wrong because his belief that in some cases there was no "material lesion" contradicted the fundamental tenet that a "physical disorder almost always precedes the moral lesion."[38] Ferrus declared that in mental illness

there is always a physical disorder that, even though in some rare cases [is] subsequent to the moral disturbance, requires no less a physical treatment . . . [and] generally precedes the intellectual disorder. If one consults the history of a disease . . . one ascertains that there had been various disturbances of sensibility before the outbreak of delirium, that the patient complained of cephalgia and of digestive disorders, slept little or uneasily, had become peculiar and bizarre, etc. Therefore, the point of departure of [mental] alienation is most commonly a physical lesion, a lesion that is not always demonstrable anatomically; yet is it not thus in many questions of medicine and ought not the inadequacy of observation be attributable to the lack of means for investigation?[39]

Ferrus also echoed Blanche's fears that Leuret's methods of intimidation were dangerous and inhuman; having witnessed Leuret's techniques many times at Bicêtre, where both men held posts, Ferrus had discontinued them. He felt that they were detrimental to the "pleasant and affectionate—though firm—discipline" of his own ward at Bicêtre; the frequent harsh words and cries from Leuret's service unsettled his own patients, he asserted. Ignoring the fact that Leuret had not advocated the exclusive use of moral treatment, Ferrus argued that if Leuret's ideas were applied generally the "intimidation method would prove to be a misfortune, and therapy would regress to the centuries of barbarism and ignorance."[40] As a final sarcastic jab at Leuret, Ferrus announced that he himself would not remain mute in the face of Leuret's assertion that his tactics ought to be employed universally,[41] an allusion to Leuret's reported attempt to cure a "voluntarily mute" thirty-five-year-old woman by simulating the patient's speechlessness.[42]

Were the allegations of Leuret's brutality true? On the one hand, his moral methods were oriented toward the particular circumstances of the individual patient and perhaps were more interventionist than those of his peers in psychiatry. His skepticism about the use of pharmaceutical preparations in the treatment of insanity led him to be more experimental with moral treatment than other physicians. This skepticism was founded on cases such as one involving a forty-four-year-old male domestic who developed suicidal tendencies and became quite agitated when he was dismissed on the death of his employer. A doctor administered sulfate of magnesium, which did not bring about a cure. Yet, after being sent to Bicêtre, Leuret cured him in twenty-one days by simply making him the caretaker of the hospital's dining hall.[43]

On the other hand, there was a darker side to Leuret's methods. He was fond of using showers to bully patients into renouncing their fixed ideas; patients were often placed in a tub of lukewarm water, and from a height of two meters a column of water was directed on their heads for five to thirty seconds. Some of the patients at Bicêtre were so afraid of Leuret's showers that it was only necessary to position them under a faucet to secure the desired concessions and disavowals of their phobias. Leuret sometimes complemented this shower with another variety of shower: the patient was stretched out on a inclined plane and doused repeatedly with buckets of cold water.[44]

Thus, there was truth in the accusations of inhumanity and barbarism leveled at Leuret. However, when his often punitive method of treatment is contrasted to the utter drudgery, remorseless routine, and blindly conventional medical therapy characterizing most French asylums of the day, the point becomes moot. If Leuret's critics rejected his views and favored what they thought was a less punitive form of therapy, they also wished to engender in the patient a strong confidence in medical authority, thereby strengthening their dominance over their patients and fostering deference toward their professional role in mental hospitals. As Michel Foucault has argued, hidden behind psychiatric claims that a particular institutional therapy represents humanitarian progress are usually agendas that seek to discipline and punish inmates more effectively.[45] Consequently, the largely hostile reaction to Leuret's ideas, though in many cases well-intentioned, may have had less to do with the barbarism associated with his therapeutic techniques than with their professional implications. Sincere concerns for patient welfare were sometimes eclipsed by powerful motives of self-interest.

The professional implications of the controversy were so distressing to some of Leuret's critics that they failed to see the subtleties of his theory. For example, Leuret had not proposed moral treatment as the only form of therapy for mental alienation. Both the academy's reporter and Leuret himself in his *Moral Treatment* pointed out that he believed that organic processes could be responsible for mental illness in some cases. Leuret rejected the allegation that his views were the same as those of the German J. C. Heinroth (1773–1843), who believed that insanity was a sin and that the moral force in human beings could never be destroyed by physical forces. For Heinroth a lunatic was morally culpable for his or her affliction. The anticlericalism of many early nineteenth-century French alienists guaranteed that Heinroth's theological version of psychiatry would not be popular in medical circles and explains why Leuret was so intent on denying the connection that some of his opponents drew between his views and those of Heinroth. The notion that human beings possessed a vital force more powerful

than the forces of physics and chemistry, according to Leuret, ignored the effect on the mind of a severe blow to the head, as well as
the ingestion of poisonous substances and the inflammation of the
brain.[46] Indeed, it could be argued that Leuret took the most sensible position that because an organic basis for each variety of mental
disorder had not been discovered, the best therapeutic approach
was to counteract the empirical affective symptoms and their patent
moral etiology with psychotherapy. By ignoring the validity of his
views and focusing instead on the issue of brutality, his opponents
eschewed science in favor of dogmatic positions that obscured the
issue that disturbed them more deeply: the theoretical and professional implications of Leuret's therapeutic approach.

The crucial point on which the controversy hinged seemed to be
whether madness was essentially a physical disorder, and on this
point the majority of the academy's doctors agreed with Dr. J.
André Rochoux (1787–1852) that "there is no insanity without delirium. . . . [B]ecause one only thinks with the brain, there can be
no insanity without a physical lesion. . . . Therefore, one ought to
admit in principle the existence of these lesions, though they are
not always perceived by the senses."[47] Without the understanding
that insanity was a somatic malady, its treatment would cease to be
an exclusively medical affair. Because Leuret had argued that the
phenomena of insanity did not conform to the "general laws of matter,"[48] it would be easy to conclude that it could be treated only by
moral means and hence that the physicalist remedies psychiatry
owed to mainstream medicine would be incidental to the healing
process.

Psychiatrists were alarmed by Leuret's views because they appeared to endorse the continued involvement of Catholic clerics in
the treatment of the insane. When Leuret's *Moral Treatment* appeared in 1840, the conflict between organized medicine and the
Church was intense. Many Catholics sought to protect the medical
activities of the religious orders in France. They attacked the monopoly of the medical profession for curtailing the freedom of
French men and women to seek cures for their illnesses wherever
they wished.[49] Physicians, on the other hand, sought to eliminate
clerical competition, a huge task in the provincial regions of the
country. In the *département* of Maine-et-Loire, for example, hospices run by Catholic nuns housed large numbers of insane men and
women. Alienists like the fiercely anticlerical Ferrus had to cam-

paign tirelessly to convince local administrators that the zeal with which the religious orders protected their jurisdiction over the mad was generally harmful to public mental health.[50] Their task was made all the more difficult because clerics who operated hospices for the insane explicitly exploited the element of religious consolation in moral treatment to justify their continued participation in the institutional care of lunatics.[51] Accordingly, alienists were intent on establishing that insanity was essentially a physical disease, for this authorized exclusive medical care of the mad. As long as people believed that the brain operated according to laws contrary to those that governed the other organs they would not accept the doctor as the sole therapeutic authority in mental pathology.[52]

Lay observers also pointed out the professional implications of Leuret's doctrine. The journalist Louis Peisse said that the question of the organic nature of mental alienation had grave practical significance, for if madness were a disease of the soul or mind, then it would not be an exclusively medical concern. Indeed, it would not constitute a disease in the medical sense, and consequently, theologians, moralists, and penologists would be entitled to treat the insane. It was little wonder, then, that the immense majority of doctors believed that insanity depended upon a "morbid state of the body . . . "; in other words, that it had its seat in the brain.[53]

Albert Lemoine, a spiritualist philosopher, expressed much the same opinions in 1862. Lemoine observed that the question of whether insanity was a bona fide disease was crucial to alienists. According to him, a doctor was essentially a "healer of the corporeal machine"; if insanity were only a derangement of the mind the physician could claim no special expertise in its treatment by virtue of his medical background.[54]

Lemoine's nonmedical status enabled him to make another trenchant observation about the rancorous infighting between the partisans of moral and medical therapy. Lemoine was struck by what he termed the truly surprising feature of the entire debate: although they all attacked each other fiercely, the "most stubborn adversaries" actually agreed without knowing it.[55] For example, manual work, exercise, or showers could be seen as either a moral or physical method.[56] The real disagreement was over the theoretical nature of insanity and its seat, Lemoine said.[57] In all practical respects, the antagonists were equivocal and far from consistent.[58] Thus, their conflict mainly took place on the level of discourse. In practice, tradition and routine held sway in most asylum wards when it came to therapy and care and, if Leuret's more tempered views of the 1840s are taken into consideration, the use of physicalist medical remedies was probably never significantly reduced even in his own ward at Bicêtre.

Unfortunately, Leuret did little to defuse the tension, conflict, and misunderstanding. On 10 January 1846 he reported to the Academy of Medicine on three cases of insanity that he had treated. One had called for an exclusively physicalist therapy, while another required a combination of moral and somatic remedies. The third, however, was a case of depression in which moral treatment alone was successful. Leuret concluded that there were no strict guidelines for the treatment of mental disorders, for "there are clues [to the proper remedy] that vary infinitely, because they depend on the nature of the patient's mind, his character, his education, his age, his sex, the form, causes and duration of his delirium, his social position, his customary relationships, and finally the character, activity, and resources of the doctor himself." These many considerations made therapy an "art, like rhetoric, painting, music, and poetry," Leuret wrote, and not a science, because they made therapy dependent on the doctor's intuition, imagination, sensitivity, and inspiration and not on professionally approved rules.[59]

It is easy to imagine how medically trained alienists would have reacted to such a notion. Even the normally sympathetic Brierre de Boismont conceded that inspiration constituted an "immense domain in which it is extremely easy to go astray" and acknowledged that Leuret's flair for popularizing his ideas made them susceptible to exaggerations and exploitation by uncritical laymen.[60] Dr. Charles Lasègue agreed and, in an obvious allusion to Leuret's January report to the academy, said that in the absence of an approved *materia medica* and a precise classification of mental diseases, many doctors, in despair at finding the cause of madness, had reacted by prescribing "the life-style that ordinarily accords the best with the health of the intelligence: a retirement home, quiet distractions, pleasant travels, a select and infrequent social life, books that are easy to read; in a word, all the conditions of life a calm and healthy-minded person would take pleasure in." But, Lasègue pointed out, this approach would merely "substitute hygiene for medicine, prophylaxis for treatment," and in instances of mental alienation it was ordinarily too late to apply preventive measures. Thus, the adherents of moral treatment erred in their responses to the admittedly incomplete state of mental pathology. Moreover, to resort to inspiration in moral treatment was unwise:

It is difficult to count on inspiration when one is free to choose neither the time [of the onset of illness] nor the subject matter; and no matter how formidable the intelligence or the resources that inspiration has at its disposal, it is never up to the task imposed on the alienist. The most persevering and active mind has its hours of discouragement and weakness; it then must rely upon a more firm support, capable of resisting the indecision of our mental faculties.

Lasègue advised against siding with Leuret or the latter's enemies who took a less aggressive approach to moral treatment; to side with either would mean perpetuating the errors of the past or disregarding what was valuable and germane in the writings of earlier thinkers.[61]

Well into the 1840s, Leuret's detractors chose to view his theories as heretical and described his therapeutic endeavors as largely ineffective. Leuret was not alone—Louis Delasiauve, who owed his appointment at Bicêtre to him, remained loyal to his ideas,[62] as did Maurice Macario, a doctor who had interned under him at Bicêtre.[63] Yet Leuret and his followers seem to have been outnumbered within mental medicine. As Lemoine wrote in 1862, most doctors were physiologists who viewed insanity as a bodily disease and regarded troubled mental faculties as only effects or symptoms of a more basic organic disorder.[64] Still, Leuret's influence was not without its consequences: as one doctor lamented in 1853, the divisive quarrels between the advocates of moral and medical therapy had led to the almost total abandonment of narcotics in the treatment of madness.[65] Such developments made many doctors uneasy, and their uneasiness was increased because during the 1840s and 1850s psychiatry was taken to task several times at the Academy of Medicine over the issue of the uncertain somatic pathology of insanity, the issue to which Leuret had helped draw attention.[66]

One form of medical response was the counterattack. Rochoux, who in the *Lancette française* had challenged anyone to present a mental phenomenon that could only be explained by psychology,[67] declared that it was wrong to suggest that there was no material lesion of the brain in insanity simply because the lesion was not detectable in many cases. In a burst of questionable reasoning, Rochoux argued that since there can be no effect without a cause, there had to be an organic lesion in order for mental alienation to strike. Madness, he concluded, must stem from a lesion of the brain or of the mind, and from the medical point of view it made no sense to say that one could treat a disease of pure mind.[68]

Guillaume Ferrus staunchly supported Rochoux,[69] but strong words were not enough to resolve the debate surrounding the somatic pathology of insanity and the effectiveness of medical remedies for the somatic lesions in mental alienation. It was François Leuret's iconoclastic theory of moral treatment that brought into the open the dangers posed to alienism by this debate. Like Pinel, Leuret criticized the use of physicalist therapies because usually signs of somatic damage in the brain could not be detected in autopsy. Leuret argued that the causes of insanity belonged to an order of phenomena foreign to the laws of organic matter: emotions and ideas. He also shared Pinel's dislike of physicalist remedies because they seemed to authorize the notion that insanity was primarily a chronic disease that the doctor was relatively powerless to cure. The Leuret episode was similar to the situation faced by British alienists in the early nineteenth century: having successfully attained some recognition of their role in the diagnosis and treatment of insanity, they confronted a growing interest in the moral therapy practiced at the York retreat by Samuel Tuke, whose ideas were similar to Pinel's. Tuke was a layman, and his writings, like Leuret's, constituted an attack on the capacity of the medical profession to deal with mental illness. Tuke's moral therapy, also like Leuret's, was designed to address the individual needs of the patient.[70]

In the French case, many alienists felt that accepting Leuret's ideas meant jettisoning their medical models of insanity and compromising their roles in its treatment, an alarming prospect for a group that had just received governmental approbation in 1838 as medical functionaries responsible for the insane in state asylums. By identifying Leuret with J. C. Heinroth, whom they condemned for his religious characterization of insanity and his advocacy of a rigorous moral treatment, French psychiatrists confirmed that their attacks on Leuret were motivated by their wish to scuttle any theory of mental disease that might justify clerical involvement in the treatment of the mad. Leuret's generally negative attitude toward the large public mental institutions authorized by the 1838 law[71] further indicated that his views were distinctly at odds with French alienism after 1838. As their British colleagues had done in response to Tuke's theories, French psychiatrists sought to defend their control over their patients and asylums in the period subsequent to the appearance of Leuret's writings. English alienists resorted to somatic and biophysical explanations of insanity to achieve this objective and a popular form of this strategy in the 1820s and 1830s was an appeal to phrenology as a way of demonstrating that the mind was an integral part of nature and biology.[72] In the second half of the nineteenth century French psychiatrists opted for hereditarian explanations of insanity like degeneracy theory. The alienist who was at the center of the controversy over Leuret's methods and who was one of the first to embrace hereditarianism as an explanation of lunacy was Jacques Moreau de Tours. His role in psychiatric affairs between 1840 and 1860 anticipated the response of his profession to the religious implications of Leuret's ideas.

Jacques Moreau de Tours and the Crisis of Somaticism in French Psychiatry, 1840–1860

The controversy over insanity's somatic pathology did more than cast doubt on psychiatry's claim that it alone was qualified to treat mental diseases. If alienists could not identify lesions for each type of mental disturbance, they were unjustified in contending that only doctors were capable of diagnosing insanity. This fundamental weakness in psychiatric knowledge meant that the psychologically oriented academic philosophers of the French university system could claim that they were no less adept than alienists at distinguishing madness from sanity, particularly in borderline instances involving apparent reason mixed with hallucinations. Thus, French alienists' occupational status during the July Monarchy and the Second Empire was challenged not only by the Catholic Church but also by the spiritualist school of philosophy. The career of Jacques Moreau de Tours perhaps best illustrates psychiatry's efforts to improve its fundamental professional interests in the face of such challenges. From 1840 to 1860 Moreau endeavored to reestablish insanity as an organic phenomenon and to certify it as an exclusively medical problem.

Moreau was born in Montrésor in the department of Indre et Loire on 3 June 1804.[1] His father was a soldier in the armies of the French Revolution and of Napoleon and received the Cross of the Legion of Honor; after Waterloo, he spent the rest of his life in political exile in Belgium studying mathematics. Moreau began his schooling in Chinon with the classics and attended the College of Tours. He spent the next two years studying medicine at the public hospital of Tours, after which he moved to Paris to obtain his medical degree. On 6 July 1826 he became an intern at Charenton, where he was tutored by Esquirol. On 9 June 1830 he successfully defended his medical thesis.

One of the methods Esquirol favored in the treatment of madness was traveling, and he often sent his students as companions for patients on extended trips. Moreau made such a trip to Switzerland and Italy. When he returned in 1836 he published a book on the influence of strong emotions on mental disease and organic affections. For the next three years Moreau traveled with another patient through Egypt, Palestine, Syria, and Asia Minor and was so fascinated by what he saw that he adopted the customs and dress of these countries, including the use of hashish.

When he returned to Paris, he obtained an appointment at Bicêtre, where, he discovered, the hospital's alienists were divided into two camps, one for and one against Leuret. Moreau, who later recounted his shock at Leuret's use of a cold *douche* to browbeat a patient,[2] quickly became one of Leuret's most vocal critics.[3]

When Esquirol died in 1840, Moreau was asked by Jules Mitivié, Esquirol's nephew, to join him and Baillarger at Esquirol's private asylum at Ivry outside Paris. In 1861 he replaced L. F. Lélut at Salpêtrière, where he worked until his death in 1884.

Moreau has been described as a lifelong somaticist.[4] But he changed his opinions about madness in 1840–1841 when he began experimenting with hashish and working at Bicêtre. It was then that he realized that all his ideas, "laboriously acquired over twenty-five years, on the true and essential nature of madness, were false and erroneous."[5] He became a member of the Hashish Club, a group of artists and writers that included Théophile Gautier. His experimental observations were published in his *Hashish and Mental Illness* in 1845, a work that provides important clues about Moreau's reasons for abandoning his earlier views.

Moreau began his studies of the effects of hashish on the mind with what he claimed was a new and illuminating method of psychological observation. He practiced self-observation by taking hashish and exploiting its capacity to produce hallucinations without destroying self-consciousness, observing through his "inner consciousness" the vivid dissociation of ideas in intoxication.[6]

Moreau believed that this method was superior to the method used by Pinel and Esquirol, who ascribed "too much importance to simple appearances" by concentrating on the varieties of psychological symptoms.[7] Pinel could be excused because, Moreau said, he was mostly concerned with devising a classification system for mental diseases and therefore observed from "too distant" and "too general a point of view."[8] Esquirol went further in exploring psychology but was content in the end to attribute mental disorder to the patient's illusions. Moreau disagreed, arguing that

there is no error, mistake, or *illusion*, except through the confusion of the judgement that is no longer in a condition to judge, to appreciate the products of the senses. One does not have an illusion (in the pathological sense of the word) because an affliction of the eyes or ears distorts images and sounds, but one truly has an illusion when, as a result of some mental disturbance, he makes an erroneous judgement.[9]

By experiencing what he alleged was the same kind of mental state as that in insanity, Moreau felt he had gained a novel appreciation of the subjective nature of madness. For example, he contended that

when any person believes that hallucinations are assailing him, we have a fact of mental pathology whose origin must be found elsewhere than in his ignorance or in his incapacity to appreciate a phenomenon with ignorance. . . . A madman believes because he believes, just as he is afraid because he is afraid; there is no other reason for acts of madness except their very fact.[10]

The first of the two principal conclusions that Moreau drew from his self-observations under the influence of hashish and from contemporaneous psychiatric literature was that "all forms, all occurrences of delirium or of actual madness, all fixations, hallucinations, irresistible impulses and so forth, owe their origin to a primary mental change, identical in all cases, that is evidently the essential condition of their existence. It is *manic excitement*."[11] The second was that psychologically there is no distinction between the dream state and the delirium experienced in both insanity and hashish intoxication.[12]

In drawing the first conclusion, Moreau was endeavoring to make a case for the organic nature of madness and hence to defend medical prerogatives in the treatment of insanity. He sought to go beyond what he described as the unedifying disagreements among physicians over mental and physical causes.[13] He wished to characterize the *"primary fact,* the primary functional lesion from which flow all the varieties of madness."[14] The nature of this lesion, whatever its causes, was organic,[15] yet Moreau recognized the great difficulties encountered in describing it accurately. He felt that psychiatrists before him had failed to shed much light on insanity because they had "sought an organic explanation for the grain of sand that jams the mental apparatus, and . . . looked ultimately to the brain cells to explain mental disorders."[16] These

partisans of the physical lesion theory, completely unable to show these lesions, as, for example, with tuberculous deposits in pulmonary consumption or the swelling of the glands of Peyer and Brunner in chronic fevers, blame the imperfections on our methods of investigation and resort to reason to establish the existence of these lesions. No functional disturbance can exist without a lesion in the organs in charge of those functions. That is unquestionable; but what do those people say who recognize only functional disturbances? So long as we have not been shown an organic lesion, we must at least be permitted to remain in doubt.

Furthermore, we should take into consideration that in many cases madness is simply a way of viewing the world that differs from the accepted one, a few eccentric, isolated ideas that have no bearing whatsoever on the collective mental faculties. When one sees certain delirium disappear as if by magic under the influence of a strong emotion, then it becomes impossible to look for organic alterations. Only the mind can be accountable for the disturbances of the mind. Has it ever occurred [to Leuret and his followers] to inquire what lesion of the brain, what arrangement of cerebral molecules, are responsible for false beliefs, erroneous ideas which we are all subject to, whether we are educated or ignorant?[17]

Moreau felt that both the strict somaticists and the spiritualists were wrong. He believed that the body was fundamentally involved in each mental disturbance but that pathological anatomy—the examination of the "inner texture of the organ"—was not the method that disclosed the physical problem. Only his hashish-induced self-observation offered the means to properly appreciate "what type of organic lesion might cause the primary fact of dissociation of ideas." This organic lesion, Moreau maintained, resulted from a change in blood circulation:

one sees from this that we too concede a functional lesion, not independent of the organs as believed by the partisans of some unknown mental
dynamism, but linked essentially to a completely organic and molecular
change, however imperceptible its nature, imperceptible as the changes
that take place in the intimate texture of a rope to which one applies
vibrating motions of variable intensity.[18]

These comments, appearing in Moreau's *Hashish and Mental
Illness* in the chapter on the use of hashish in therapy, suggest that
he may have been using the example of hashish's physiological effects on the mind to undermine Leuret's argument that mental
illness could be treated psychologically, that is, as if it did not necessarily coincide with an organic lesion of the nervous system.[19] This
would help to explain why *Hashish and Mental Illness* ended
abruptly with the section on hashish in therapy and why Moreau
admitted that his experience administering the drug led to no firm
conclusion concerning its effectiveness.[20] The editor of the modern
edition of *Hashish and Mental Illness* hypothesized that Moreau,
rushing to submit it for a competition sponsored by the Academy of
Medicine, had failed to finish the book. Yet, whatever the explanation, Moreau's treatment of hashish as a curative tool was perfunctory. Committed to disproving the notion that mental patients could
be cured by reasoning alone, he was more interested in establishing
the somatic nature of insanity's fundamental lesion than in exploring methodically the use of hashish in the treatment of madness.

Moreau's argument that mental disturbance in insanity was essentially caused by a failure in blood circulation was also curious.
He wrote that when the hashish experimenter felt the "manic excitement" at the onset of delirium and heard the "bubbling sound
which coincides with mental disturbances," he would recognize the
similarities to the psychological phenomena observed in "congestive ruptures, falls or blows on the head, hemorrhages, the inter-
ruption of periodical bloodletting, the action of certain nervous
stimulants such as alcohol, Indian hemp, opium, and in general of
all narcotics." In all these states of mental derangement there were
"almost certain signs of a disturbance originating in the blood-
stream." Because of its similarity to other psychological disorders
triggered by physiological conditions and linked to circulatory dis-
ruptions, Moreau confidently affirmed the somatic nature of mental
alienation.[21]

However, Moreau's argument, based on analogy and little else, was weak. It is debatable whether self-observation could confirm that an essentially organic process was responsible for all varieties of madness. As one critic has pointed out, Moreau's experimental approach was vulnerable to the charge that a purely subjective perspective necessarily altered the nature of the mental phenomenon to be observed.[22] Charles Lasègue's position on the matter in 1846 was probably the most balanced: while admiring Moreau's talent and intellectual audacity, he could not agree that Moreau had successfully equated the psychological state of madness with the mental state of hashish intoxication.[23]

These weaknesses in Moreau's argument suggest that he was intent on addressing issues not immediately apparent without a consideration of the professional and intellectual context of the times. His insistence that insanity's "primary fact" was an entirely organic phenomenon indicates that he was attempting to bolster psychiatry's image as a medical specialty that ministered to the mind through the brain. He himself was aware of this image and wrote that even his opponents within psychiatry, who viewed madness as a primarily psychological malady, were obliged periodically to consider the physical phenomena of mental disease because "being doctors, they are compelled to do medicine, however little they do it."[24]

It is not surprising that Moreau was an advocate of physicalist therapy. In his thesis (1830) he had written that "the most important part of the treatment of mental alienation" was the elimination of the "idiopathic or sympathetic cerebral affection" by methods of counterirritation and anti-inflammation, such as bleeding, purgatives, and the use of quinine sulfate. This approach, Moreau asserted, was founded on physiological laws and on therapeutic practices supported by more than thirty years of psychiatric experience.[25] In the 1840s and 1850s Moreau published extensively on experimental treatment with toxic substances of mental disorders such as hallucinations, melancholy, and intermittent insanity.[26] His experimentation with a wide range of medicinal properties suggests that Moreau never wavered in his belief that it was the body to which alienists ought to administer their remedies. To have thought otherwise would have been professionally calamitous, as Moreau acknowledged in 1851, and would have meant ceding the therapeutic initiative to lay psychotherapists or "ministers of religion."[27]

The second of the two conclusions Moreau drew from his obser-

vations in *Hashish and Mental Illness* was that dreaming and
insanity were identical processes, and here too he was intent on
justifying professional prerogatives. This conclusion was also characterized by odd lapses in scientific thinking. For example, Moreau
had inferred from the resemblance between the stimulation of
memory and imagination in hashish intoxication and in dreaming
that madness and dreaming were psychologically identical,[28] an in-
ference that provoked criticism even from colleagues who believed
that insanity and dreaming were highly similar. Moreau had written
that the dream state occurring in madness was one of a "sleepless
dream, where sleep and the waking state are mingled and confused."[29] Jules Baillarger argued that this hypothesis made little
sense, for if mental alienation was a "mixed state resulting from the
fusion of the sleeping and waking state," then how could the dream
and insanity be identical? "Is it not impossible," he asked, "for a
state that is comprised of two opposing conditions to be identical
with one of these two?"[30]

Moreau continued to cling to his theory despite the cogent criticisms of Baillarger and a number of physicians at the Academy of
Medicine.[31] Such tenacity suggests that he was motivated by more
than disinterested scientific reasons. By maintaining that insanity
was psychologically identical to dreaming, alienists could argue that
hallucinations were always involuntary—and hence pathological—
phenomena, for in many French intellectual quarters dreams were
held to be absolutely devoid of rational meaning. Therefore, in the
interpretation of mental states of questionable pathological status—
such as hallucinations without apparent psychological derangement—lay opinions would have to defer to medical diagnosis.

Psychiatry's main competition in the diagnosis of hallucinations
came from academic philosophy. Throughout the July Monarchy,
Victor Cousin dominated university philosophy with his doctrine of
"eclecticism," renamed "spiritualism" in the 1840s. Among other
things, Cousin's eclecticism taught the existence of God, free will,
and the spirituality and immateriality of the soul. According to Laurent Cerise, Cousin's teachings constituted a "psychologism" that
upheld the primacy of the ego, reason, and the individual conscience.[32] Cousin also taught that the most fundamental mental
phenomena could be understood through introspection, that is, the
examination of one's own psychological functions through reflec-

tion. In its stress on individual freedom and the reconciliation of diverse intellectual traditions—such as Protestantism and Catholicism—eclecticism was the philosophic counterpart of an Orleanist liberalism that sought to live in peace with the Church. Indeed, as the foremost member of the Royal Council of Public Instruction between 1830 and 1850 Cousin was a powerful political figure, and it is not surprising that alienists worried about their diagnostic prerogatives. Psychiatry's claims to expertise were threatened by French academics' argument that to distinguish between sanity and madness it was necessary to refer to the psychological laws governing the normal functioning of the mind, laws that psychologists alone knew. This contention helped to shape Moreau's thinking on the relationship of insanity to dreams.

Once again Leuret was at the center of the controversy with his argument that insanity was basically an exaggerated error in thinking and that reason was the standard for judging whether an individual's hallucinations constituted a mental illness.[33] He alleged that the customary medical criteria for distinguishing reason and madness were inadequate, especially with regard to the "mixed state" of genius and apparent madness in the same person, and concluded that if the varieties of obsessional delusions and fixed ideas encountered in a typical asylum were used as the criteria for judging insanity, it would be difficult to identify anyone as sane. Similarly, if alienists were to institutionalize all persons who retained consciousness of their hallucinations, virtually everyone would end up in a mental hospital. Leuret advised alienists to fall back on what passed for knowledge of the laws governing the functioning of the healthy mind in order to make the distinction between an insane and normal idea.[34]

Leuret's point of view carried with it, however, the professionally disadvantageous suggestion that medical expertise by itself was insufficient for accurately measuring the pathological extent of a deviant affect. According to Brierre de Boismont, Leuret's theories were "victorious proof of the advantages of the intervention of philosophy in medicine." How could doctors pretend any longer that a vast gap separated philosophic questions from practical and applied medical matters? Brierre de Boismont believed that psychiatrists were still best qualified to deal with philosophic questions about mental alienation,[35] but by conceding that madness was a field of inquiry to which philosophy could make crucial contributions, he implicitly endorsed the intervention of nonmedical interests in the study of aberrant mental phenomena.

An ominous sign of the threat posed to psychiatrists by nonmedical intervention occurred at the Academy of Medicine on 8 April 1845 when Dr. Frédéric Dubois d'Amiens argued that the different views of insanity held over the years by Cullen, Pinel, Gall, Broussais, and Esquirol could not explain mental disease. It was necessary, he said, to go beyond their physiological and pathological notions to the psychological perspective because "doctors did not render a sufficient account of the psychological facts" of madness. Dubois concluded that only the psychologist could distinguish a reasonable individual from a mad one. For example, physicians could not explain how in hallucinations and dreams the mind experiences many bizarre sensations without the organs of sense providing it with external stimuli. What, then, distinguished the case in which a sane person hallucinated from a case of complete insanity with hallucinations? Dubois maintained that the organic school had no answer to his question; only the psychological school could supply the criteria with which the difference between reason and madness could be identified. The principal criterion for Dubois was simple: one was sane if one did not believe in the reality of one's hallucinations. The same thing applied to dreaming: because the ego was often aware of dreaming in the dream state, it could not be a pathological condition.[36]

Dubois's central and psychiatrically heretical argument was that the diagnosis of madness was best left to someone who had examined carefully the many functions and phases of mental life, including dreams and hallucinations. Defending the medical point of view, Guillaume Ferrus took Dubois to task for separating disorders of the mind from dysfunctions of the body. He objected that there was no reason for treating questions regarding the pathology of the brain differently from questions of pathology regarding other organs because in all diseases it was the functional disturbances that revealed the disorders within the somatic animal economy. There was no need, therefore, to appeal to philosophy, for its "systems" invariably encouraged errors regarding the nature of mental illness.[37]

Ten years later psychiatry still had not silenced calls for nonmedical intervention in the diagnosis of insanity and for the need to employ psychology to complement mental medicine. In 1851 the philosophy section of the Academy of Moral and Political Sciences announced an essay competition on the topic of the psychology of sleep. L. F. Lélut, an alienist and member of the academy, for the most part was unimpressed with the entries, as were other physicians, including Laurent Cerise. Cerise complained that instead of undertaking serious studies of all aspects of sleep, the authors had restricted their investigations to petty questions: for example, what happened to the "faculties of the soul" in sleep and how were they modified? Cerise remarked that such questions were enough to disillusion any physicians who might have naively believed that the academy's program appealed to medical knowledge and experience. Cerise also declared his impatience with the "metaphors of literary language" employed by the psychological school, expressions such as "the soul feels this or that" or "reason combats, submits to, accepts. . . . "[38] Lélut was hardly more generous. He castigated Albert Lemoine, the author of the winning essay, for his spiritualist belief that the soul was pure, unalterable, and ultimately independent of the organs.[39]

There were good reasons for an alienist to be wary of Lemoine. An orthodox spiritualist philosopher, Lemoine made clear his belief that the psychological approach differed substantially from the medical one with respect to the anomalies of mental life such as madness, drunkenness, fever, and dreaming and that a psychologist was capable of explaining all varieties of mental phenomena. Philosophy could become a "medicine of the soul," he argued, and in this endeavor it was wiser to refer to the "reason of the sage" than to the "delirium of the lunatic" in order to determine whether someone's mental state was diseased.[40] For Lemoine, the key to understanding the "different alterations" of the mind and body during sleep, disease, madness, drunkenness, hypnosis, and ecstasy was the normal state of the waking and the healthy body and mind.[41] For the physician, he admitted, there was always a distinct difference between health and illness in all these states because a physician only saw an organic change. The psychologist, in contrast, saw no fundamental difference between normal thinking and mental dissociation because the soul, although temporarily crippled by the "blind and capricious influence of the body," never suffered an essential change. The psychologist, Lemoine argued, saw only differences in degree. He was willing to grant that the body's organs could be diseased in madness, but he believed that the mind or soul expressed itself in ways that deviated from normal psychical operations and had nothing to do with strict pathology.[42] In effect, Lemoine warned doctors to leave the interpretation of psychopathology to psychologists and concern themselves exclusively with the study of the diseased body, as Dubois had warned them in 1845. Lemoine felt—and his opinion was obviously shared by other nonmedical figures—that alienist expertise could not distinguish morbidity on the basis of mental symptoms alone. Yet to restrict doctors to the study of diseased organs was hardly acceptable to psychiatry, the branch of medicine that had the most trouble correlating symptoms with physical lesions.

The incompatibility of medical and psychological interpretations of phenomena such as hallucinations that seemed to occupy the middle ground between normal and pathological thinking was clear by midcentury. The tension between psychology and alienism had been building for about thirty years, a period that had witnessed quarrels among psychologists, metaphysicians, and physicians, disputes that created a "great noise" in the French scientific world.[43] In 1862 Lemoine termed these quarrels a virtual war between doctors and philosophers-psychologists, resulting in the separation of the professions with little exchange of ideas.[44] Psychologists suspicious of psychiatry took pleasure in pointing out its glaring weaknesses. As Lemoine wrote:

since the physiologist does not find any further characteristic difference between the corporeal conditions of a madman and a man of reason who errs, he must at least ask of psychology what distinguishes simple error— compatible with the possession of reason—from insanity or delirium. . . . If medicine rashly rejected the insights of psychology . . . it would thus omit the capital element of madness—the disturbances of the mental faculties—the one truly consistent symptom that reveals the existence of the organic disorder.

How could a physician distinguish a reasonable idea from an insane notion when the somatic pathology of madness was clouded in obscurity? Lemoine asked.[45]

Alienists came under fire for their construction of psychiatric syndromes such as insanity with reason (*folie raisonnante*) and insanity with conscience (*folie avec conscience*), in which the patient was conscious of the morbid nature of his fixed ideas. These syndromes constituted a major problem for alienists, who had to demonstrate that consciousness of one's own illusions did not disprove the absence of free will and hence the involuntarism crucial to the diagnosis of mental alienation. For the alienist Jules Falret, the task for psychiatry was to apply the clinical method of examining the full variety and sequence of physical and mental symptoms in the same patient over time. To do otherwise, Falret continued, was to defer to psychologists, moralists, and magistrates. Insanity without apparent delirium was a variety of madness that "men of the world, philosophers, and magistrates" viewed as simple eccentricity or originality of character. It was hardly surprising, then, that alienists were accused of inaccurate diagnosis in cases of madness with reason, Falret concluded, and only the careful application of a method based on the clinical observation of pathological symptoms in conventional asylums could show that certain people who at one time might appear sane would at another time display the delusional thinking and behavioral abnormalities of outright madness, thus vindicating psychiatric diagnosis.[46]

In midcentury France there was a strong current of resistance to alienists' attempts to distinguish sanity from insanity on the basis of purely mental symptoms. State university philosophers who, even after Victor Cousin's fall from power in 1850, remained loyal to Cousin's spiritualism, continued to reject medical interpretations of psychological phenomena that seemed to suspend the powers of the rational will. Hallucinations were the principal phenomenon to engender controversy between alienists and Cousin's followers, and it was widely recognized that the dream constituted the key to discovering the laws governing hallucinations. From this perspective, Moreau's interest in the relation of madness to dreams is understandable, but what did his belief that they were identical have to do with the professional challenge that academic philosophy posed for psychiatry?

In his *Hashish and Mental Illness*, Moreau had acknowledged the diagnostic problems presented by the "almost infinite variations of delirium" and the consequent "caution shown by most authors in attributing delirium to an organic lesion."[47] Hallucinations seemed to similarly defy pathological diagnosis, and their ability to occur without the mind being truly injured buoyed "those who want to see in psychosis only a functional disturbance, a psychic change that has nothing to do with lesions of the mental organ. . . . The psychotic would mainly be an individual with a special point of view, whose thoughts differ *in form* but not in intrinsic nature from those of other men." Moreau set out to demonstrate that hallucinations, "even in cases where the integrity of the mental faculties seems intact," were the product of "a general but rapid and instantaneous disruption of these same faculties." The similarity between insanity and the regression and dissociation of the mental operations in dreaming led him to argue the "hallucinations that seem to coexist with an unquestionable state of mental health must be classified with other phenomena of mental illness."[48]

Why should Moreau refer to the ostensibly normal mental function of dreaming to establish the pathological status of hallucinations?[49] The answer lies in a consideration of the prevailing philosophic milieu. Moreau borrowed his notion of a dream-psychosis identity mainly from Maine de Biran (1766–1824), the philosopher instrumental in shaping the doctrine of spiritualism.[50] The similarities between the dream state and insanity had been observed by others before Maine de Biran; Cabanis, for one, had cited them in the early 1800s.[51] But Cabanis believed that the mind conserved a part of its activity in sleep and dreams. Maine de Biran did not. He held that sleep was completely ruled by organic functions, that the mind was entirely passive under these conditions, and that sleep was the domain of absolutely involuntary mental and physical life, a state of animal existence identical to insanity. Consequently, dreams were nothing but the result of "organic dispositions" of cerebral matter. Maine de Biran categorically denied that thoughts in dreams could be meaningful or attest to the presence of reason or divine inspiration; he restricted freedom of the will entirely to the waking state so as to protect it from "sensualist" philosophers who viewed even the state of health as the product of "organic movements."[52]

Maine de Biran drew a solid line between the mental activity in the waking and sleeping states. Moreau, too, held a low opinion of the psychical functioning in dreams: for him dream-thinking and freedom of the will were mutually exclusive.[53] By adopting Maine de Biran's ideas, Moreau had succeeded in arguing that the study of psychology had nothing to do with the question of sleep. J. A. Rochoux recognized this feature of Maine de Biran's doctrine; he wrote in 1846 that the French philosopher—although "the most insipid, emptiest and most impotent of retrograde metaphysicians"—had substantiated the medical view that the phenomena of pure psychology ceased with the onset of sleep.[54]

By drawing on the work of Maine de Biran, Moreau had made a strong case for banishing psychologists from the diagnosis of the diseased mind and for the identical nature of the mental states of dreaming and insanity. Hence, a hallucination, whether it occurred during sleep or in the waking state, was always involuntary and pathological. The expertise of a physician was therefore essential to the interpretation of hallucinations coexisting with an apparently sound mind. As Lemoine observed in 1862, the philosophy of Maine de Biran had placed the insane beyond the jurisdiction of psychology and squarely in the hands of medicine,[55] which is certainly where Moreau wanted it to be. As he had written to his friend Alfred Maury in 1845, his *Hashish and Mental Illness* had been composed to refute the conventional view that madness ought to be defined only in terms of the healthy state of the mind's faculties.[56]

Moreau's exploitation of Maine de Biran's ideas could easily be interpreted as calculated. He had cited the authority of an influential contemporary philosopher whose complete works had recently been published under the editorship of Victor Cousin.[57] It could hardly be coincidental that Maine de Biran's ideas had been brought to the attention of the psychiatric community in 1843 with the publication in the *Annales médico-psychologiques* of A. Royer-Collard's "Examination of Maine de Biran's Doctrine on the Relationship of Body to Mind in Man."[58] Moreau was a contributor to the journal, and it is unlikely that he was unaware of this article. Nor did Moreau simply borrow the notion of an identity between dreams and insanity; his method of self-observation under the influence of hashish sounds suspiciously like Maine de Biran's method of introspection that allegedly disclosed the principles of mental functioning.[59] Moreau nowhere acknowledged a debt to Maine de Biran, but it is hard to believe that he was not influenced by Maine de Biran's philosophy. Therefore, it is likely that he borrowed some of Maine de Biran's ideas in order to embellish a professionally advantageous theory. In the process, he called into question the competence of academic philosophy to identify the limits of disease and sanity in hallucinatory mental states.

Still, Moreau's theory of dreams and his ongoing efforts to dem-

onstrate that insanity was a physical malady met substantial opposition throughout the 1840s and 1850s. This resistance to Moreau's
ideas, as well as the cognitive uncertainty within the profession and
the shakiness of its claims to exclusive treatment and diagnosis of
mental disease, was vividly illustrated at the meeting of the Academy of Medicine on 8 May 1855. The meeting was convened to
hear the report of Jean Baptiste Edouard Bousquet (1794–1872) on
Moreau's paper "On Madness from the Pathological and Pathoanatomical Point of View."[60] Bousquet's report and the ensuing discussion were obviously of great interest to alienists, filling sixty-five
pages of the *Annales médico-psychologiques* in 1855. Moreau himself seems to have taken special notice of this debate, for he essentially repeated his argument regarding dreams and insanity from
Hashish and Mental Illness in the same volume of the *Annales*.[61]
The recent and largely nonmedical analysis of the subject of sleep
at the Academy of Moral and Political Sciences also doubtless inspired him to republish his ten-year-old thesis.

The meeting began with Bousquet's scathing attack on mental
medicine and Moreau's paper. Moreau had sought to prove that
insanity, despite its unquestionably exceptional characteristics, was
not essentially distinct from other illnesses of the brain. Moreau
found the comparison with neurological disorders such as hysteria
and epilepsy to be apt: in these diseases, he stated, there is a common and "primitive" lesion of "nervous dynamism" that was identical to the functional lesion found in cases of insanity. By going beyond the symptomatological level and postulating a fundamental
nervous lesion responsible for psychoneuroses, neurological disorders, and psychosis, Moreau felt justified in equating delirium and
madness. This notion, he conceded, flew in the face of the received
ideas of his day. However, he argued that in as much as it strengthened the connection between insanity and other diseases of the
organism, it enabled physicians to counteract their alleged therapeutic powerlessness that stemmed from the prevailing indecision
over the pathological nature of insanity.[62]

Although not all doctors of mental medicine agreed with
Moreau, Bousquet saw much in Moreau's thinking that reflected
the typical attitudes and ideas of the alienist community. He accused alienists like Moreau of using delirium as an important part of
their definition of insanity.[63] This was a mistake, Bousquet main-

tained, for the differences between delirium and insanity far out-
weighed their similarities. For example, delirium occurred ordinarily with fever and general functional disturbances, while insanity
often struck people in otherwise perfect health.

Bousquet also objected to Moreau's notion that madness
stemmed from a lesion of the brain. He granted that the brain was
the "material condition" of thought but denied that the cause of the
disturbance in the brain's activity during mental disease always re-
sided in the brain, as Moreau believed. Bousquet cited a number of
venerable theorists, including Cabanis, Pinel, and Esquirol, who
had written that often the origin of insanity was in the reproductive
organs or in the viscera.

Moreau's explanation of the absence of pathoanatomical lesions
in autopsies of the insane satisfied Bousquet even less. Moreau had
written that a structural lesion frequently disappeared in the transition from the acute to the chronic stage, a process that accounted for
the negative findings of so many postmortem examinations. To
Bousquet this was merely another expedient employed by psychiatrists for half a century to explain away the absence of organic lesions of the brain's tissues. How, he asked, could one continue to
believe in these lesions when the "testimony of the senses" indicated that the proof of these "material brain alterations" was beyond
demonstration?

Bousquet next criticized Moreau's hypothesis that all forms of
madness and delirium were produced in a mental state identical to
sleep.[64] If this were true, he reasoned, it meant that every night
almost everyone went mad only to recover sanity upon waking. Yet
if there was no insanity without a cerebral lesion, the same had to be
true for the state of sleep. This could not be, he concluded, because
it was inconceivable that a disease that stripped human beings of
their "noble attributes" and terminated in death in many cases
could be such a "light" and transitory condition. It was incorrect to
press the analogy between sleep and madness, according to Bousquet, and it was definitely a mistake to equate them.[65]

Bousquet's criticisms were hard to refute, Louis Peisse observed
two years later.[66] Equally galling for psychiatrists was that his criticisms closely resembled those Leuret had made fifteen years earlier.[67] Bousquet, like Leuret, sought only to characterize the state
of mental pathology at the time and to dispel all notions not based

on the strict observation of the phenomena. Noting Moreau's defense of psychiatry's therapeutic competence, Bousquet challenged him to show how his somaticist orientation had led to new and better treatments.[68]

Bousquet's report sparked responses from a number of the academy's physicians. Ferrus and Baillarger jumped quickly to psychiatry's defense. To Baillarger, Bousquet's comments suggested that both the classification and observation of mental illnesses since Pinel's day had led to nothing more than a cognitive chaos, which the mental asylums reflected. However, the better part of Baillarger's protest was directed at Bousquet's refusal to accept the theory that a material lesion was the cause of insanity and the therapeutic consequences of such a theory; here the relation between the somatic pathology of mental disease and the therapeutic profile of alienists became clear. By casting suspicion on Moreau's efforts to demonstrate that madness was a disease of cerebral "organization," Bousquet had "spiritualized" madness and depicted it as an illness of the soul, Baillarger maintained. In the process Bousquet had endorsed Leuret's moral treatment of reasoning and words. "Why," Baillarger asked, "compare the struggle between the doctor and his patient to a discussion of philosophy and morality" as Leuret and Bousquet had done?

Baillarger also addressed Bousquet's criticisms of the psychiatric fondness for pointing out the similarity between madness and sleep. Baillarger restated his own theory that the principal condition of dreaming was "automatism," the involuntary exercise of the mental faculties that also served as the "point of departure" and basis of delirium and madness.[69] This theory of mental automatism was virtually identical to Moreau's theory of involuntary psychical regression during the mental excitement of dreams and can also be traced to the work of Maine de Biran.[70] By basically agreeing with Moreau and Maine de Biran on the psychological similarities between dreams and insanity, Baillarger also sought to establish that the mental operations in madness were solely the concern of a physician.

Baillarger called Bousquet's criticism of psychiatry "heresy."[71] Another physician referred to it as "blasphemy."[72] There is no mistaking the perception of some psychiatrists that Bousquet's remarks were professionally subversive. Ferrus was surprised that Leuret's views could have resurfaced to rekindle "the same [old] arguments, the same controversies." Bousquet, warned Ferrus, was saying that insanity was a nonmaterial disease and that "medicine has been, is, and will be constantly powerless to cure it" unless it employed "purely moral means."[73] And when given a chance to reply to his opponents, Bousquet did accuse psychiatry of therapeutic "poverty" and accused alienists of feeling satisfied with their occasional ability to confirm the diagnosis of incurability because it relieved them of the responsibility to cure the illness.[74] According to Bousquet, "of all the aspects of mental pathology, therapeutics is . . . the least advanced: it is the most important and [yet] that which leaves the most to be desired."[75]

From the comments and reactions of the academy's psychiatrists, it is plain that the 8 May meeting brought into the open the problems that had been plaguing mental medicine for twenty years. Bousquet had drawn attention to the often dubious way in which many psychiatrists had compared madness with dreams in order to confirm the pathological nature of hallucinations. He also repeated the claim voiced more than once by the proponents of moral treatment that some alienists too often resigned themselves to therapeutic pessimism because of an unwillingness to view insanity as anything but a somatic disease. To a physician like Ferrus, Bousquet's advocacy of moral treatment as a solution to this dilemma threatened the exclusive therapeutic prerogatives of psychological medicine, as Leuret's theories had fifteen years before. According to Ferrus, clerical interference in the treatment of madness still threatened psychiatry in 1855; he looked forward to the day

when the therapy of [mental] alienation has achieved its independence of action, its free scope; the day when it has ceased to be a tributary of idealist and theological beliefs; the day when a famous prelate, persuaded by our arguments has recognized that madness could be elucidated only by medicine and reason; the day, finally, when medicine itself could say: "Alienation is a disease like all the others."[76]

There is no reason to doubt the sincerity of Ferrus's conviction that the realization of all these hopes would benefit the mentally alienated immensely; nonetheless, there is equally no reason to doubt that he and his colleagues Moreau and Baillarger hoped that these developments would also bring concrete professional advantages.

It is also evident from the remarks of Bousquet that Moreau
reflected the views of a good many French alienists in his treatment
of madness and dreaming as well as the somatic pathology of insanity. Stymied by the failure to correlate organic lesions with the wide
range of psychical states accompanying mental alienation and the
failure to establish firm clinical criteria with which to identify madness, alienists had been compelled to explore new ways of elu-
cidating the nature of insanity. Some, like Moreau, probed the
problems of madness by exploring the phenomenon of delirium.
Moreau compared the dreamlike delirium of his hashish hallucinations with the delirium of fever, cerebral congestion, other narcotics, and excessive cold, thirst, and hunger. Because all these states
of delirium were so similar and were plainly caused by pathophysiological changes in the body, Moreau hoped to demonstrate that
every hallucination was the result of a somatic process in the cerebrovascular system.

Moreau must have realized that the opposition to his ideas drew
strength from pointing out that his argument was based only on
analogies and circumstantial evidence, for beginning in the early
1850s, he produced a series of papers on the influence of heredity
in mental pathogenesis. In the naturalist and biological phenomenon of heredity Moreau believed he had finally found the organic
component in madness for which he had been searching for almost
twenty years, the somatic missing link that would prove that only
doctors of psychological medicine were entitled to diagnose and
treat insanity. He started with mental pathologists' frequent observation of a mixed state of hallucinations and clear reason in certain
persons. In 1845 Moreau described how the phenomenon of hallucinations without apparent mental disorder had encouraged thinkers like Leuret to reject the notion that there were organic lesions
of the brain in insanity. In 1850 Moreau conceded that reason and
madness could not be distinguished absolutely, yet he asserted that
there was one "fact of pathophysiology" that explained the mixture
of these two states in one person: heredity.[77] By studying the gene-
alogy of an individual who exhibited this curious psychological condition, he declared, one would find that the person's ancestors and
descendants manifested either the mixture of madness and genius
or one of the two exclusively.[78]

In a paper read to the Academy of Medicine in 1851, he repeated his theory that in all the cerebral disorders of madness and beneath all the moral and physical causes that engendered them, there was a "pathological fact, a dynamic nervous lesion."[79] This lesion was expressed by a functional disturbance of the vital force inherent in the organization of the nervous system, a force Moreau called *névrosité*. He attributed this lesion of nervous force to the hereditary transmission of the nervous system from parents to children, citing as evidence studies that argued that there were laws governing the hereditary transmission of entire organ systems in animals.[80] According to Moreau, this meant that insanity was a "pure and simple nervous affection," produced by the inheritance of a faulty nervous system.[81]

Moreau brought together his ideas on heredity in his *Morbid Psychology in its Relationship to the Philosophy of History* in 1859. For him heredity was the key to explaining the relation of affective phenomena to the organs of the body and to explaining how someone could be mentally ill despite appearing to be rational at times.[82] Human reproduction was the biological truth that succeeded where the pathoanatomical and psychological viewpoints had failed, supplying the unmistakably organic condition for the great variety of deviant mental states.[83] It helped to undermine "the moral theories of insanity that gain credence so easily in the world, and against which even great medical minds are not put sufficiently on guard."[84] It also accounted for the automatism evident in hallucinatory and dream states, for these involuntary mental functions were produced by the psychocerebral "excitement," whose physical source was a hereditary neuropathic condition.[85]

So important was the pathological factor of heredity for Moreau that he claimed it could be regarded as a lesion in itself.[86] It served as a highly successful somatic point of reference with which he felt he could explain virtually all the troublesome phenomena of morbid psychology. Heredity to Moreau was particularly relevant as a clinical concept because, he claimed, its influence was far more pronounced in pathology than in the state of health.[87] Moreau cited Claude Michéa, another alienist, who in 1852 had identified heredity as a diagnostic principle that enabled doctors to distinguish between "morbid perversion" and nonpathological moral failure.[88]

Moreau's treatment of the issue of morbid heredity was not without its difficulties, however. He proclaimed that 164 out of the 192 cases he had examined showed a distinct physiognomic resemblance between the insane patients and their parents.[89] But Moreau's study had rested on the initial diagnosis of his insane patients, whose pathology he had deduced from their abnormal psychological complexes. To show that heredity was a major factor in mental pathology Moreau had had to assume the very thing that had to be proven: the pathological nature of certain deviant mental states. To demonstrate that insanity was a somatic phenomenon by referring to heredity, he was compelled to base his conclusions on cases in which the only symptoms were psychological. Moreover, in what would become a familiar refrain for psychiatrists studying the hereditary effects of insanity, Moreau admitted that there were at least two serious problems associated with his inquiries: the necessary information about family members was often hard to obtain and the testimony of his patients was unreliable. Finally, the appreciation of physiognomic resemblances was almost as subjective a process as the interpretation of morbid psychology: similarities in brain shape between patients and parents were hard to establish precisely, which left the way open for prejudice to influence opinion.

Despite these difficulties plaguing Moreau's "scientific" studies of morbid heredity, there were good reasons for citing the role of hereditary predisposition in mental alienation. During the 8 May meeting of the academy, Baillarger, Ferrus, and P. A. Piorry all invoked heredity as a somatic factor that contradicted Bousquet's advocacy of moral treatment and his criticism of the psychiatric belief that insanity was organic in nature.[90] To Ferrus, nothing proved the "material conditions of madness" more than heredity, which clearly involved the physical organism.[91] The inheritance of physical and mental features implied that the organism was fundamentally involved in the transmission of characteristics from one generation to the other. Thus, if madness were inherited, it was a certifiable disease of the body and was treatable with the irritants, tonics, sedatives, and purgatives that asylum physicians continued to use throughout the nineteenth century.[92] For example, P. A. Piorry (1794–1879), who wrote an influential book on heredity in 1840, believed that the organic disposition to insanity was inherited through the blood.[93] Because most of the medical therapies of the time were designed to counteract hyperemia of the brain and stabilize cerebrovascular conditions,[94] Piorry's concept of heredity did nothing to contradict the therapeutic orientation of alienists or the popular notion that madness was a disease of the blood. Nor did Moreau's theory that changes in blood circulation caused mood disturbances: if insanity were the result of a hereditary neuropathic condition that ultimately concentrated in the brain—which, Moreau explained, was "irrigated" by more blood and retained less blood than any other organ except the lungs[95]—then remedies that affected vascular conditions would be appropriate in its treatment. Consequently, Moreau's hypothesis of a significant hereditary dimension to mental alienation entitled psychiatrists to continue to employ their conventional medical remedies in the treatment of insanity and strengthened the argument that symptoms of questionable morbid status were the result of distinct pathophysiological conditions and were the exclusive province of psychiatry.

The medical credentials of psychiatry were enhanced by a strategic appeal to the physical approach, "the fixed centre of psychiatry" that links mental medicine as an occupational group to the rest of medicine;[96] and underlying this process was the issue of professional autonomy.[97] In the middle third of the nineteenth century French psychiatry confronted the threat of clerical interference and criticism from the philosophy professors of the Sorbonne. It also confronted elements within medicine whose skepticism of psychiatry's claims to positive knowledge of insanity fueled lay criticisms. Moreau's career and the development of his ideas between 1840 and 1860 reflected the professional aim of French alienism to eliminate nonmedical competition from the analysis of deviant mental states and the treatment of the mad.

Moreau's hereditarian approach to mental disease was a pioneering one, and acclaim was not long in coming. In 1859 Dr. Maximin Legrand praised Moreau's *Morbid Psychology* for answering the questions of psychology by examining the "diseased organism."[98] In 1860 B. A. Morel also applauded Moreau's efforts to amplify the importance of hereditary insanity.[99] By the time of Moreau's death in 1884, hereditarianism had become the main diagnostic orientation of French psychiatry. His striking exploitation of morbid heredity as a theoretical concept in the 1850s heralded this dramatic development in the intellectual history of nineteenth-century French psychiatry.

Chapter Four

Alienism and the Psychiatric Search for a Professional Identity: The Société médico-psychologique, 1840–1870

The psychiatric move toward hereditarianism was caused by other factors than simply those relating to the treatment and diagnosis of insanity. Sociopolitical disorder affected the efforts of the alienists of the *Annales médico-psychologiques* to organize a learned society of psychiatrists between 1843 and 1852. The political events of 1848–1851 interfered with alienist attempts to professionalize through association and were responsible for the clerical reaction that marked the first decade of the Second Empire (1852–1870). To ensure the success of the first psychiatric society in French history, alienists had little choice but to accommodate themselves to the new regime and the changed cultural conditions after 1852. Because of its repeated assertions of social usefulness and philosophic and religious orthodoxy, the fledgling Société médico-psychologique helped to improve relations between mental medicine and the state. Yet medical willingness to strengthen its ties with the imperial state in order to assure the continuity of psychiatric practice in public asylums meant that alienism ran the risk of being identified with the government and hence of becoming a vulnerable target for critics of Louis Napoleon's administration. When public attacks on alienism mounted in the 1860s, asylum psychiatrists began to formulate a hereditarian model of mental disease calculated to convince the imperial government of their expertise and to postpone official inquiries into alienist practice.

Plans for the Société médico-psychologique began when alienists affiliated with the *Annales médico-psychologiques* expressed their desire to form a learned society of psychiatrists. Jules Baillarger was the first to propose such a step. In the first issue of the *Annales* in 1843 he noted that English alienists had already founded an association of asylum doctors and had met twice, on 2 November 1841 and on 2 June 1842. Baillarger recommended following the English example by meeting annually to discuss the treatment of madness and asylum management, hygiene, and construction. Baillarger believed that the insane of France could only benefit from the improved therapy and care that would result from the collaborative efforts of psychiatrists. He also foresaw the advance of medical science, because with annual meetings alienists could agree on specific topics that they could study according to common guidelines. He believed that with this kind of concerted effort great theoretical breakthroughs were likely.[1] In the July 1843 issue of the journal Baillarger referred to his planned association of alienists as a *société médico-psychologique*, the name that eventually was accepted officially.[2]

For the next two years the project attracted little attention. However, in the September 1845 issue of the *Annales médico-psychologiques* the young alienist B. A. Morel wrote an open letter to Guillaume Ferrus from Italy, where he had been observing the treatment of the insane. He expressed the wish that French alienists found "a medical society, whose goal would be the study of everything that relates to the pathology and physiology of the nervous system, as well as the improvement of insane asylums." Morel hoped that a new psychiatric association would keep abreast of foreign publications dealing with the same issues.[3]

Interest in Baillarger's project began to mount in 1846. In the March issue of the *Annales médico-psychologiques* Baillarger reaffirmed his original plans, concluding that the comprehensive study of mental illness was feasible only if a medical association was founded. The same year Emile Renaudin and Honoré Aubanel, asylum doctors at Fains and Marseilles respectively, wrote to Baillarger in support of the plans for an alienist association; their letters were published in the *Annales*. Aubanel in particular praised Baillarger's ideas and echoed the desire for an official group of doctors working together to solve problems such as those presented by the legislation concerning public assistance to the insane. He thought

that the initiative for such an association would have to come from
Paris because of the geographic isolation of so many physicians in
France. He proposed that a medical congress be held there under
the auspices of the inspector-general of the public asylum system
and the minister of the interior in order to decide upon the guidelines for the new medical society. Finally, he agreed with Baillarger's and Renaudin's vision of an alienist association as an agency
for compiling statistics on asylum admissions and discharges and the
incidence and causes of madness. [4]

Statistical studies were very popular among French doctors at
midcentury, especially in the Paris region. [5] Psychiatric statistics in
the nineteenth century tended to be inconclusive and generally
provided few concrete findings, yet no one suggested that they be
abandoned. It is likely that psychiatrists of the time compiled statistics because they anticipated that this activity would bestow "a
sense of scientific legitimacy" on their fledgling profession. [6] It was
also politically expedient for a group of doctors intent on forming a
socially useful psychiatric association to appear as scientific as possible. Accordingly, after noting that the success of such a "vast enterprise" as the formation of the Société depended on the approval
of the government, Baillarger added that the primary goal of the
new society would be to "publish statistical research conducted according to a uniform plan." [7]

The eagerness of Baillarger, Morel, Aubanel, and Renaudin to
form a new psychiatric association was understandable in light of
the news that in addition to the establishment of a British society for
the improved care of the insane in 1841, asylum doctors in the
United States had also formed an association in 1844. Alienists were
responding as well to the restless spirit within French medicine in
the 1840s and the importance of "association" in post-1815 French
society. Doctors were not alone in seeking a professional identity
and solidarity through organization; school teachers, lawyers, and
civil servants also struggled to gain status on the basis of their supposed expertise. French physicians sought legislation that would
raise standards of training, eliminate competition from unlicensed
healers, and improve public confidence in organized medicine. [8]
Dissatisfaction with the state of medicine had prompted doctors to
convene the national medical congress of 1845 and publicize their
grievances. They hoped that a collective and official protest would

encourage the minister of public instruction to meet their demands, thereby improving their social standing.[9]

Alienists especially believed that "association" would benefit their branch of medicine. The editor of the *Annales médico-psychologiques*, Dr. Laurent Cerise, though not an alienist himself, had written that because of the dramatically changed and largely unregulated social and economic conditions of early nineteenth-century France, doctors were at a disadvantage unless they embraced the principle of association. His argument echoed similar ones then being heard throughout France. Socialists and defenders of the working class like Cerise's mentor Philippe Buchez promoted association as a way of increasing labor's political power and safeguarding the interests of workers.[10]

However, plans to form a psychiatric association would not be realized for another two years, during which time Baillarger's professional authority grew substantially.[11] With his entry into the Royal Academy of Medicine in Paris on 15 June 1847, the Salpêtrière doctor could successfully overcome the skepticism and indifference of some psychiatrists and assure the civil authorities of the alienists' good faith. In the January 1848 issue of the *Annales médico-psychologiques* Baillarger announced that on 18 December 1847 the decision had been reached to form the Société médico-psychologique. Now that the English alienist Dr. Forbes Winslow had followed the example of the *Annales* and begun *The Journal of Psychological Medicine and Mental Pathology*, Baillarger wrote, it was appropriate that French doctors emulate their colleagues in Germany, England, and the United States by forming a psychiatric association of their own. He called for a society that united the physicians whose careers were devoted to the study and treatment of insanity and the "physiologists, administrators, savants, jurists, moralists, and philosophers" whose writings contributed to an understanding of psychology.[12]

The statute of the Société médico-psychologique was published in the same issue of the *Annales médico-psychologiques*. Its themes and objectives were bold and broad. It stated that medical science could no longer be restricted to its traditional sphere, for it was tied unavoidably to "considerations of a higher order, relative to religion, morality, jurisprudence, education, metaphysics, administration." Mental pathology was a crucial part of medical science. Its study raised many of the most profound questions of philosophy and social science and underlined the importance of the physiology and pathology of the nervous system for these disciplines. The preamble to the statute called for the end of mental pathology's "fatal separation" from other fields of knowledge. The authors of the preamble believed that as a forum for midcentury psychiatrists the Société médico-psychologique would contribute decisively to the solution of some of the most refractory social and philosophic problems of the day.

It was also clearly stated that while the Société would continue to mirror the interdisciplinary ethos of the *Annales*, the most constructive contributions to an understanding of psychology would come from the medical members. The society would be structured to ensure medical hegemony. Of the five sections stipulated in the preamble, the first two—mental pathology, and the anatomy and physiology of the nervous system—were to include only physicians. This amounted to one-half of the society's forty-eight resident members, that is, those who lived in the department of the Seine. Each of the other three sections—moral hygiene, legal medicine and the administration of madness, and philosophy from the perspective of the relationship of body to mind—consisted of eight resident members, of whom at least two had to be physicians. Consequently, there would always be more doctors than laymen within the resident Société médico-psychologique.[13]

Although it could be said that the Société was a logical and practical consequence of the *Annales médico-psychologiques*, the Société was clearly intended to be a predominantly alienist enterprise. Its founders were psychiatrists, its membership was to be chiefly medical, and its sole objective was "the study and perfection of mental pathology." If morbid psychology was seen as fundamentally related to the psychological sciences, the implication was that physicians would be foremost in any endeavor to answer questions of the functions of the mind. Moreover, the eagerness with which Baillarger and others sought to establish the Société demonstrated that they viewed it as an important step toward the legitimation of psychiatry's professional status and corporate identity. Alienists like Renaudin and Aubanel wanted the Société to be more than simply a medical learned society; they wanted it to become "a kind of interest group" that would work to improve salaries, pensions, hiring practices, and working conditions for alienists.[14] By 1848 the original group centered around the *Annales médico-psychologiques* was moving aggressively to become a medical specialist organization.

The January 1848 issue of the *Annales médico-psychologiques* included the announcement that the list of the Société's members would be published in the March issue after authorization by the Ministry of Public Instruction. However, revolution broke out in February 1848, and toppled the government of King Louis Philippe, disrupting administrative procedures and preventing the Ministry from officially approving the new Société. When the March 1848 issue appeared belatedly, the readers of the *Annales* were informed that "great political events" had proven to be impediments to its publication and to governmental approval of the Société. As the editor of the *Annales* remarked more than a century later, the Société had been a "stillborn victim" of the 1848 Revolution.[15]

It was not until March 1852, following Louis Napoleon's coup d'état of December 1851, that the Société médico-psychologique was established. Its first meeting was held in Paris at the Faculty of Medicine on 26 April 1852. Ferrus was chosen to be the first president, testimony to his status as one of the most important alienists in France at midcentury. Pierre-Nicholas Gerdy (1797–1856) was named the first vice president, Amédée Dechambre (1812–1886) the first secretary-general, Alexandre Brierre de Boismont the first secretary-treasurer, and Claude Michéa the first archivist.

Michéa, Dechambre, and Edouard Carrière (1808–1883) formed a committee to report on the changes to be made in the organization's previous statute.[16] The new statute, which turned out to be quite different than the earlier one, began by stating that political unrest and scientific progress were incompatible. This statement explained why the Société médico-psychologique had waited four years until the demise of the Second Republic to emerge as a bona fide scientific organization. By publicly denouncing the republican regime created by the February 1848 revolution, the founders of the Société demonstrated that they were anxious to align themselves with the Bonapartist Second Empire and distance themselves from the liberal-socialist alliance that had overthrown the July Monarchy.

There were other indications that the new Société was eager to make its peace with the imperial state. Michéa, Dechambre, and Carrière declared that the original statute had expressed narrow views, an inappropriately professional esprit de corps, and a medical "exclusivism" ill-suited for the new Société médico-psychologique's pledged goal of "a rapprochement between the natural and moral sciences." The psychological element in the vital sciences had been overshadowed by "physiology" in the original preamble, they continued, resulting in the general acceptance of mental phenomena as little more than the consequences of somatic functioning. Recalling the original declaration that nonmedical fields of knowledge had much to gain from medical science, Michéa, Dechambre, and Carrière objected that it was too often forgotten what contributions empirical psychology could make to the study of the physiology and pathology of the nervous system. They announced that in the new Société psychology would reoccupy the position of importance it had traditionally held in the human sciences. To underscore the promise to shed the Société's exclusively medical image, the commissioners welcomed members from philosophy, law, history, the arts, and even the clergy.

As a further blow to the medical character of the Société médico-psychologique, the commissioners abolished the five sections into which the resident membership had been divided in 1848, explaining that it was impractical to divide its small membership (thirty-five members in 1852) into sections. However, they added, even if size were not a problem, the sections would have been ultimately counterproductive, for they would have meant placing restrictions on the executives' freedom to admit new members. The implication was clear: at such a delicate stage in its history the Société's executive committee wanted to be free to accept as members those it deemed to be ideologically and professionally desirable. For example, it did not wish to be forced because of inflexible regulations to admit a physician when the acceptance of a nonmedical member would have been more expedient; article 5 of the "Conditions of Admission" stipulated that the proportion of doctors to nonphysicians would not be fixed, as it had been in medicine's favor in the 1848 statute.

Finally, the report reaffirmed that medical science touched on matters of a higher order and that the study of madness raised a number of social and philosophic issues susceptible to medical solutions. But in a passage that had not appeared in the 1848 preamble, the commissioners recognized that there were "facts of a superior order" that ought not to be omitted from the human sciences. The "active or voluntary element" that existed in "a mysterious alliance" with cerebral matter would no longer be reduced to "encephalic physiology" but would be viewed as one of the two discrete components comprising the dual nature of human beings.

Clearly some of the principles of the Société médico-psychologique had changed between 1848 and 1852. The commissioners responsible for the new statute had dropped the original regulations guaranteeing medical hegemony, probably because they feared that a pronounced medical image based on the anticlerical physiology of Cabanis, Bichat, and Broussais would be a liability in securing ministerial approval for the new Société. They preferred instead to be as conciliatory as possible by committing the Société to the goal of a rapprochement between psychological medicine and spiritualist academic philosophy and by acknowledging the relevance of "empirical" (nonmedical) psychology to understanding the pathology of the nervous system. They also accepted the notion of a free will or soul linked indissolubly to the organic matter of the brain without being a mere effect of cerebral functioning. In other words, to gain governmental sanction the Société conceded a major principle of spiritualist philosophy and Christian doctrine: the voluntary capacity of human beings to govern their own behavior and thinking. It also conceded that academic philosophy might make important contributions to the elucidation of mental illness—a considerable concession for a profession that for years had battled with official philosophy to establish that it alone knew how to tell madness from sanity.

The effort of the Société médico-psychologique to appear conciliatory and loyal to spiritualist ideas had its origin in the ideological climate of the post-1848 clerical reaction, which lasted until the early 1860s.[17] Catholicism enjoyed renewed cultural and political influence, mainly because of the Falloux law of 1850, which gave religious orders the right to open schools without any further qualification and introduced councils with strong clerical elements to control the lay university. The changed political and religious climate proved uncomfortable for academic philosophers like Paul

Janet, Jules Simon, Emile Saisset, and Adolphe Garnier, followers of Victor Cousin, who had fallen from power along with the July Monarchy. These defenders of the French university had been attacked by Catholics in the 1840s for their alleged secularization of postsecondary education. Nevertheless, in as much as they believed that human actions could not be reduced to the laws governing the physical world—as Janet put it at the Société médico-psychologique on 30 November 1863[18]—they were much more acceptable company than positivist physiologists. As Cousin himself maintained, his philosophy taught "the spirituality of the soul, the freedom of man, the law of duty, . . . divine providence, and its immortal promises inscribed in our most intimate needs, in its justice, and its goodness."[19] He argued that the sense organs were essentially instruments for the voluntary soul.[20] Cousin, an Orleanist liberal during the July Monarchy, wished to live in peace with the Catholic Church. He wanted, as the literary critic Charles-Augustin Saint-Beuve remarked, to create a great school of philosophy that "would not give offense to religion."[21] After 1852 liberal academics continued to profess spiritualist ideas because it made them appear "irreproachable to Catholics."[22] Most subscribed to a moderate republicanism based on a distrust of the clerical tendencies of Catholic churchmen, but they distinguished between the often troublesome political meddling of clerics and the theological content of Catholicism. At the same time they tried to dissociate themselves from more contentious aspects of their ideological past. For example, some Sorbonne professors emphasized their intellectual orthodoxy by rejecting the introspective method of self-observation in psychology that had characterized pre-1848 philosophy and that Catholics had attacked as self-indulgent egotism. During the Second Empire they embraced a less subjective form of psychological observation which, Janet told the International Alienist Congress in Paris on 10 August 1867, avoided the search for causes, stressed a more empirical appreciation of facts, and shed light on mental disorder in a way self-observation never could.[23]

It is no surprise that Garnier and Janet, two of the more prominent spiritualist academic philosophers at midcentury, were elected members of the Société médico-psychologique in 1854 and 1858 respectively and served as its president in 1862 and 1867 respectively. The institutional response of alienism after 1852 had much in common with their chastened spiritualism and muted republicanism. Well aware that the 1848 Revolution had made the mere existence of the Société a cause for political suspicion, alienists sought to renounce their associationist beginnings and avoid the stigma of republicanism by rejecting physiological theories of the relationship of body to mind, which had often been identified with republicanism and liberalism in the 1815–1848 period.[24]

Alienists had been as guilty of holding physiological theories as any group of physicians, reinforcing the anticlerical reputation of physicians and the battle lines between asylum doctors and the Catholic clergy.[25] Because of their vocal anticlericalism and secularism, many alienists were viewed as allies of the republican historian Jules Michelet, whose literary war against the Catholic Church in the 1840s had prompted talk of a "renaissance of Voltairianism."[26] According to lay member Alfred Maury, the Société médico-psychologique of the early 1850s had a significant number of anticlerical and republican members, such as Moreau and Louis Calmeil.[27] Therefore, by repudiating physiological theories of mind-body interaction, the Société could improve its relations with the Catholic Church and the Bonapartist regime, which initially sanctioned clericalism. This was a particularly important consideration for the alienists who had founded the *Annales médico-psychologiques* and the Société, for the *Annales* had been accused in 1846 of being openly anti-Catholic.[28]

There was some truth to this accusation. Alfred Maury and the alienist L. F. Lélut had defended the physiological theory in the 1840s that anyone who suffered from hallucinations—including Catholic saints and religious visionaries—was suffering from nervous insanity.[29] This theory not only exacerbated the quarrels between physicians and academic philosophers but also angered Catholics and orthodox alienists like Alexandre Brierre de Boismont. After 1852 most alienists must have thought that Brierre de Boismont's approach was professionally sensible even if privately they had reservations about it. In the second edition of his book on hallucinations (1853) Brierre de Boismont defended the Catholic religion, while declaring himself a spiritualist who believed that "facts in the domain of psychology have a mode of being [that is] completely different from those in the physical domain."[30]

Dr. Louis Delasiauve, a founding member of the Société, was

almost obsequious in his attempt to demonstrate the religious orthodoxy of the new psychiatric association. The 1791 law on professional associations had forbidden physicians to organize as an occupational group in pursuit of common interests and had seriously curtailed their rights to meet. The idea of association was politically controversial particularly after 1851 because it had been championed by many socialists and radical republicans during the July Monarchy. Delasiauve therefore had to proceed cautiously; in his account of the early years of the Société he blatantly tried to show that the Société was compatible with the religious spirit of post-1848 France. Acknowledging that associations had been a cause for suspicion among civil authorities for a long time, he argued that when charity and science combined, as they did in the Société, this suspicion was unwarranted. The Société's members were pledged to the humanitarian and progressive ideals of the 1838 asylum law, he wrote, and were also inspired by "pure intentions" and "productive zeal." He reminded his readers of Christ's words, "Where two or three are gathered in my name, there I am in the midst of them," which, he said, applied to a scientific organization like the Société because of its commitment to truth. Delasiauve suggested that scientific associations were more socially useful than the academies of France—a subtle barb aimed at those bastions of liberal and anti-Bonapartist sentiment—and stressed alienism's relevance to other social questions of law, penitentiary hygiene and discipline, education, and morality. By proclaiming the Christian spirit of the Société and the utilitarian role psychiatrists could play as state functionaries, he built his case for the value of the Société to the regime. His case was apparently fairly convincing, for Delasiauve's article appeared in the *Gazette hebdomadaire de médecine et chirurgie,* a journal published under the auspices of the Ministry of Public Instruction.[31]

Another indication of the Société médico-psychologique's endeavor to cooperate with the imperial state and defer to the renewed Catholicism of the 1850s was the influence exerted within its ranks by Philippe Buchez and his followers. It would be hard to exaggerate Buchez's importance in the Société. Félix Voisin (1794–1872) described him as its "principal founding member."[32] His chief disciple, Laurent Cerise, also had a large role in the founding of the *Annales* in 1843 and of the Société in 1852. Other founding members of the Société who could be considered Buchez's followers were Auguste Ott (1814–1903), C. E. Bourdin (1815–1886), Edouard Carrière (one of the three commissioners who drew up the statute of 1852), and Marcellin-Emile Hubert-Valleroux (1812–1884). Ulysée Trélat and Gerdy were also close friends of Buchez, as was B. A. Morel, for whom Buchez had secured the post of chief physician at the Maréville asylum in 1848.[33]

Buchez's stature in the Société médico-psychologique had both a practical and a symbolic importance. His past efforts to forge an intellectual reconciliation between progressives and the Catholic Church may not have pleased many Church officials during the July Monarchy, but it worked to his favor in the 1850s among the Société's members, whose pronounced ideological and professional differences surfaced during discussions of controversial phenomena of mental pathology and of general questions, such as the influence of civilization on the incidence of mental alienation.[34] As Alfred Maury observed in his memoirs, doctors like J. B. Parchappe too often lacked "a spirit of conciliation" and "disinterest," and physicians frequently allowed their personal and scientific disagreements to assume a tone of "asperity" and "brutality" at the Société. Buchez, in contrast, displayed a refreshing disinterest that Maury, although opposed to many of his ideas, admired. Adolphe Garnier was also "animated by a great desire for conciliation among the diverse philosophic schools" represented at the Société.[35] Maury himself also preferred reconciliation to the bitter disputes that characterized French medicine at midcentury.[36]

The symbolic importance of Buchez's presence at the Société was just as great. He shared the eagerness of many of the Société's alienists to renounce their pre-1848 activities and make public peace with Catholicism. Buchez had flirted with Saint-Simonianism and socialism as a young doctor and in the 1820s he had played an important role in the founding of the French Carbonari movement, a revolutionary sect dedicated to the overthrow—by violence if necessary—of the Restoration. In 1848, supported by moderate republicans, he was appointed first deputy mayor of Paris and then president of the Constituent Assembly. He was present on 15 May when the Paris mob invaded the assembly, an episode that frightened many moderates and hastened the swing of the February revolution from the left to the center. After his arrest in December

1851 during the Bonapartist coup d'état Buchez retreated from politics. His Catholicism had been growing more orthodox since the election of Pius IX as pope in 1846.[37] His polemics against Victor Cousin's ego psychology—the unofficial philosophy of the doctrinaire school of politics, which enjoyed power during the July Monarchy—were still fresh in Catholic minds, as was his participation in the Catholic educational freedom campaign that culminated in the Falloux law of 1850.

Thus, Buchez's post-1848 apolitical position, his devout Catholicism, and his longstanding denunciation of Cousin's philosophy as Protestant[38] made him a valuable addition to the Société. Not every alienist in the Société shared Buchez's views, but few articulated their objections. To alienists Ulysée Trélat, Louis Delasiauve, Félix Voisin, Prosper Lucas, and others who had been politically active republicans in 1848, Buchez's presence in its ranks could serve as signal to the Bonapartist regime of the society's political and religious orthodoxy.

According to Maury, Buchez's followers at the Société médico-psychologique, including Morel and Ott, were spiritualists.[39] As was evident from Brierre de Boismont's work, this philosophic doctrine was not necessarily inconsistent with the organicist outlook of psychiatrists. In his address to the Société on 26 July 1852, Buchez reconciled the spiritualist belief in metaphysical moral freedom with the medical view that mental illness was caused by a diseased organism. He conceded that in insanity the lunatic was deprived of free will; the patient's mind, dominated by somatic functions, was the "dupe" of the hallucinations that characterized its delirium. Nonetheless, Buchez argued, the absence of free will during intervals of insanity caused by diseased organs was not an indication that "moral liberty" was destroyed entirely or that it was of the same nature as the "organic forces" that ruled involuntary life. Free will, a force no less real or powerful than organic force, was tied indissolubly to the organism but was not simply a product of it. Free will and the organism constituted the "double nature of man." Free will was an ultimately independent "principle of activity" of a purely spiritual nature.[40]

A similar effort to prove that the medical view of insanity was compatible with belief in free will was made by Léon Rostan, professor of clinical medicine at the Paris *Faculté* and spokesman for the organicist doctrine in mainstream medicine. Rostan acknowledged in the 1864 edition of his *On Organicism* that doctors were readily accused of materialism and atheism because they were concerned only with the diseased organs and functions of the body. In a section of the book that did not appear in the 1846 edition, Rostan denied such accusations, arguing that by concentrating on the somatic conditions of disease doctors recognized that only the body could be sick, not the soul or mind. The admission that the ultimate nature of the soul was uninfluenced by the physiological conditions of insanity was "a new proof" of its immortal and "immaterial" nature, Rostan claimed. [41]

The comments of Rostan and Buchez indicate that French physicians were anxious to show that their medical orientation was not atheistic and did not rule out the possibility of a metaphysical and rational soul that ruled supreme during periods of mental health, even if it was suspended during periods of insanity. Their doctrine of a human "double nature" of immaterial mind and material body—which held that the mind could not function without the body but was ultimately independent of cerebrosomatic organization—was intended to reassure theologians that they did not challenge the existence of free will or the soul.

It was also a doctrine that the opposing schools of physiology and psychology could agree on, thereby providing hope that mental medicine could reach a compromise with academic philosophy. It served as a rallying point for medical and nonmedical thinkers interested in psychological deviance and was an integral part of the Société médico-psychologique's ideology during the Second Empire. According to the alienist Emile Renaudin, medicine had long been plunged in a conflict between materialists and spiritualists, but by the early 1850s he could detect a tendency toward a synthesis of materialism and spiritualism into a doctrine that recognized the reciprocal influence of body and mind while rejecting the reduction of one to the other. [42] According to Albert Lemoine, a follower of Victor Cousin, the Société had contributed to ending the "war" waged by physiologists and psychologists throughout the first half of the nineteenth century. He thought it especially promising that physicians had taken the first step toward an understanding of the mind based on academic philosophy and medicine. [43] In 1857 Louis Peisse also hailed the Société and its program of reconciliation between medicine and lay psychologists. Claiming that Descartes had severed what in classical philosophy had been joined together, the body and mind, he saw the founding of the Société as a hopeful sign that both mental and physical phenomena would soon be studied as fundamental parts of one "science of man."[44]

These sentiments were echoed by Dr. Eugène Billod in December 1869. He reminded his colleague Dr. Eugène Dally that the Société's goal was to "place a hyphen" between philosophy and medicine and to enlist both disciplines in the study of the same problems. Philosophers and doctors ought not to constitute two "distinct churches," he argued, for there was not "the least incompatibility between the branch of medicine we cultivate and the study of philosophy. Most of the doctors of this Société are versed in philosophic studies. It is even probable that it is the taste for these same studies that determined the choice for most of us of a specialty that is intimately tied to philosophy." Billod specifically cited the valuable philosophic insights of members Paul Janet, Maury, and Peisse.[45] Robert Hippolyte Brochin, the Société's president in 1868, also felt that its attempt to reconcile philosophy and medicine had a salutary outcome. He boasted that there were no "exclusive somaticists or psychologists" among the society's members, an inaccurate statement that nevertheless reflected the mood of many alienists and laymen within the Société.[46]

These thinkers saw no advantages in reducing one branch of knowledge to the terms of another. They felt that both disciplines could coexist independently while working together constructively. This compromise represented an important breakthrough for alienism, which, after challenging and being challenged by lay psychologists for almost fifty years, was beginning by the 1860s to be recognized by the Sorbonne as a bona fide field of expertise.

There were also signs that the efforts of the Société médico-psychologique to become ideologically palatable to the imperial state were being rewarded. The ties between the French state and the alienist profession had been cemented originally with the 1838 asylum law. Under the Second Empire the relationship became closer. Beginning in 1860, Georges Haussmann, the prefect of the Seine, made plans for a major expansion and renovation of institutional facilities for the insane. Working with the alienist Henri Girard de Cailleux—with whom he had collaborated in 1851 in the building of the Auxerre asylum—Haussmann oversaw the construction of the Paris mental hospitals of Sainte-Anne (1867), Ville-Evrard (1868), and Vaucluse (1869). These asylums were part of Haussmann's rebuilding of Paris during the Second Empire and were constructed with a view to the security of the Bonapartist regime.[47] They were also evidence that the government saw psychiatry as a corps of functionaries that could perform valuable services for the state.

Because alienists were gaining favor in imperial eyes, they were entrusted with duties that occasionally took them outside the asylums. One notable example of this was the delegation of psychiatrists sent under Dr. Augustin Constans to the Alpine village of Morzines in 1861 to study an outbreak of nervous ill health. Villagers had been suffering from recurrent convulsions and hysterical seizures, leading the local population to believe that they were in the grip of demonic possession. Posing as "epidemic fighters" determined to stamp out the natural causes of this "moral contagion," the doctors suppressed the epidemic by dispatching most of the victims to hospitals and replacing the local clergy with the help of "a small detachment of infantry and a brigade of gendarmerie." This action—authorized by the central government—was testimony to alienists' willingness to function as "medical police" in order to make psychiatry indispensable to the state.[48]

In recognition of alienism's service to the state and its ideological orthodoxy, the Ministry of Public Instruction officially named the Société médico-psychologique an association of "public utility" on 11 December 1867. This gesture of administrative approval crowned the efforts of the Société to erase medicine's reputation as a republican, anticlerical profession and to remove the stigma of association by cultivating the image of a scientific research center run by medical civil servants pursuing humanitarian goals within the national asylum system. By embracing the ethos of disinterested science, the Société may have been following a deliberate strategy to placate the Bonapartist regime for, as Maury noted in his memoirs, Louis Napoleon—whom Maury came to know while editing the emperor's history of Julius Caesar—preferred Frenchmen to pursue science because he thought that the "culture of science" was not as politically subversive as the arts.[49] Yet no matter how deliberate or conscious the intellectual change undergone by the Société between 1848 and 1867, it had been the 1848 Revolution and the subsequent political instability and strife that had forced psychiatry to drastically revise its plans to associate. When the Société opened in 1852, it was in a political and cultural climate vastly different from that of pre-1848 France. The changes after the revolution compelled alienism to temper the liberal and professional objectives it had formulated in the heady days of the previous decade and helped to shape its perception that revolutionary conditions and medical science were antithetical.

By the late 1860s the alienists of the Société médico-psychologique had reason to be wary about the consequences of sociopolitical disorder for organized medicine. They remembered all too well how a revolution had overturned the attempts of their young profession to come to terms through collective action with its socioeconomic problems. The new regime ushered in by the failed republican experiment of 1848–1851 had demanded sacrifices and ideological concessions from mental medicine. The Société's alienists ultimately benefited from these compromises, but the price exacted from the profession was high. The Société turned its back on republicanism and gradually became staunch defenders of the political status quo. In the process, the interests of alienism became identified with those of the imperial state. During the liberalization of the empire in the 1860s, the alienist doctors of the national public asylum system were to pay dearly for this accommodation with the Bonapartist regime, leaving them even more convinced that they were social pariahs and innocent victims of popular mass movements.

Chapter Five

French Alienism and Antipsychiatry, 1860–1900

Just when it seemed that the Société médico-psychologique's policy of accommodation would solve psychiatry's political problems, mental medicine was confronted with an antipsychiatric campaign launched by the French press after censorship laws were relaxed in 1861. Newspapers of every political stripe questioned the therapeutic usefulness of lunatic asylums and accused alienists of complicity in the hospitalization of innocent people, triggering a series of ineffective legislative attempts to revise the 1838 law. Even some physicians cast doubt on psychiatric competence. Alienists reacted by debating the intellectual and institutional foundations of their profession. As the criticism continued, many psychiatrists came to see themselves as a beleaguered group surrounded by a society that did not appreciate the scientific value of their professional activity, the complexity of mental disease, or their managerial function as custodians of the mad.

While the fortunes of the Société médico-psychologique were improving by the end of the Second Empire because of its conciliatory policy, psychiatry as a whole was facing a new threat. In the wake of the war with Italy in 1859 and the Anglo-French commercial treaty of January 1860, Louis Napoleon began the liberalization of his regime, which included a series of decrees in 1860–1861 mitigating the severity of the press laws of 1852. With censorship eased, French newspapers quickly focused on mental medicine as a convenient target for indirectly attacking the Bonapartist government.[1] According to one member of the Chamber of Deputies, the imperial government was not unhappy to see the journalistic campaign against alienism because it distracted public attention from more overtly political issues.[2] Alienists found themselves in the unenviable position of bearing the brunt of anti-Bonapartist sentiment, apparently with the tacit approval of the government. The impact on French alienists was almost immediate: in 1864 B. A. Morel reported that as a result of the public hostility toward psychiatry a malaise had gripped the branch of the medical profession that delivered public assistance to the insane.[3] This antipsychiatric campaign did not begin to abate until the Franco-Prussian War of 1870–1871 and persisted in a slightly less virulent form until the end of the century.[4]

One of the earliest contributors to the antipsychiatric campaign was Dr. Henry de Castelnau, a member of the Société médico-psychologique. In two lectures delivered at the Paris Academy of Medicine on 12 July and 23 August 1859, Castelnau announced his objections to article 489 of the Napoleonic Code, which stipulated that someone diagnosed as insane could lose the legal right to administer one's own affairs and to have children. It seems that this measure was enforced frequently, for 113 of the 557 patients at Charenton had lost these rights as of 5 December 1863. Their rights were supposed to be restored when their illness was cured. But, according to Castelnau, in a recent six-year period there had been 3,201 such interdictions and only 137 reversals of the same decision—a recovery rate of only one for every 23.38 cases. This suggested to Castelnau not only that individual rights and liberties were threatened but also that an insane asylum was not an effective therapeutic institution. He alleged that despair overwhelmed the majority of committed patients, with the result that mortality rates were very high for the first twelve months and the cure rate unimpressive for subsequent years. In addition, the interdiction process encouraged families to try to profit from the misfortune of their hospitalized relatives and to then forget about them.[5] As one doctor said, without a better chance of cure there was little reason for even a concerned family to maintain interest in a committed relative; family members soon ceased visiting and eventually authorized the director of the asylum to reduce the daily pension of the patient, making the prospect of cure even more remote.[6] In response to such unflattering observations about his profession, the asylum psychiatrist Henry Bonnet remarked that Castelnau's attack on the interdiction process could easily "degenerate" into "a formal indict-ment" of the medically approved method of isolation in an asylum.[7]

Daniel Brunet, medical director of the Dijon asylum, agreed with Castelnau and painted a bleak picture of the asylum system and the regulations of the 1838 law. Because of the recent attacks on asylum psychiatry it was not the most appropriate time to criticize the 1838 law, he admitted, but he believed that the law left the insane at the mercy of their families and gave too much admin-istrative power to medicine. He said that a medical certificate did little except condemn someone to perpetual confinement, charging that the interests of the mad were not safeguarded by the visits of the magistracy and public prosecutor to the asylum because "these visits are almost always illusory" or perfunctory. When patients complained about the conditions of their confinement, Brunet con-tinued, their petitions were sent to the asylum medical director, who had no interest in conducting an inquiry. Brunet concluded that because the departmental prefects, the Paris Prefecture of Po-lice, and asylum doctors were too powerful, the insane were mis-treated frequently and people with marginally disordered thinking could be hospitalized as dangerous to society.[8]

The principal charge leveled against the alienist community was that mad-doctors were responsible for arbitrarily hospitalizing French citizens in insane asylums. It was charged that such unjust institutionalizations occurred because private asylum doctors were much too prompt in declaring a person insane, notably when to do so would add another paying pensioner to their lists of hospitalized patients.[9] This did not apply to public asylum doctors, however, because the state allottment for each inmate was inadequate to cover the costs of housing a lunatic. Instead, critics depicted the public asylum doctor as an accomplice of the state in its ongoing endeavor to preserve social peace and eliminate its opponents by incarcerating them in insane asylums.[10] This allegation had surfaced in 1837 during the debates over the proposed legislation for the national asylum system, when the political opposition accused the government of creating new ways of imprisoning political ene-mies.[11]

What was particularly distressing for alienists about the antipsy-chiatric campaign was that they were attacked by newspapers of both the left and right. Criticism of the 1838 law had "becom[e] the darling of the liberal press" by the mid-1860s. This mystified alienists like Louis Delasiauve, who could not understand why the liberal press would ally with the clerical party to malign a profession that in his eyes represented science and progress.[12] The psychiatrist Henri Dagonet observed that in order to destroy the legal provisions for hospitalization and the network of national asylums, newspapers representing religious and monarchist interests had allied with the newspapers of the "democratic party." Of course, Dagonet added, once the ruin of the asylum system had been achieved, the different factions would again go their respective political ways. Catholics would be only too happy, he alleged, to transform psychiatric hospitals into "cloisters" and to reinstate a "medicine of the soul" based on the belief that insanity was a sin and best treated by a priest. But he confessed his surprise with the liberal and democratic newspapers and cited the article by the Voltairian Louis Jourdan in the 12 December 1864 *Le Siècle* that reported that of the thirty to forty thousand hospitalized lunatics in France, fifteen to twenty thousand were the victims of arbitrary confinement. Jourdan charged that it was the 1838 law and not a real increase in the number of madmen that was responsible for the doubling of the hospitalized population of the insane between 1836 and 1864.[13] Théophile Rousselin, another alienist, also remarked on the alliance between newspapers such as *Le Temps* and *Le Siècle* and Catholic groups that sought "the radical reform" of mental institutions. He accused the political newspapers of filling impressionable minds with absurd ideas: for example, that the 1838 law violated the principle of individual freedom; that the insane were more effectively treated in their own homes; that asylums were "factories of incurability"; and that each asylum was a "Bastille" in which a citizen could be interned solely on the basis of a medical certificate.[14]

With more voices raised against the power of psychiatry and the specter of wrongful confinement, ex-patients began to submit petitions to the French senate protesting the treatment that doctors gave in asylums. The petition that started the wave of formal complaints was penned in 1864 by Aline Lemaire, a nurse at the Châlons-sur-Marne mental hospital. She echoed the standard litany of asylum horrors: doctors reigned supreme in the asylums, indefinitely confining patients, ignoring their complaints, and punishing them when they failed to conform to behavioral standards. In short, she declared, patients were at the mercy of a profession that wielded absolute power within the walls of the mental hospital. Her petition was supported by *Le Monde*, *Le Temps*, and the proclerical *Journal des villes et des campagnes*, which carried her 19 January 1864 letter to the editor protesting the "medical omnipotence" of psychiatry.[15] The discovery by an administrative inquiry that her petition had been largely inspired by the asylum chaplain, who disliked the medical director, came as little surprise to alienists who already suspected that much of the opposition to psychiatry was clerical in origin.

Similar allegations of psychiatric neglect and malfeasance appeared in newspapers such as *La Presse* and *Opinion Nationale*. Doctors were accused of being "ignoramuses" who constituted a "school" that had not progressed since the days of Molière. "Science," some antipsychiatric writers had declared, "does not value individual liberty." Alienists reportedly incarcerated scores of innocent people in prisonlike hospitals. Psychiatrists were supposedly also agents of a law that operated arbitrarily and had been devised to fight social deviance. If some considered the post-1838 asylum to be a modern version of the Bastille, others felt that the medical certificate authorizing institutionalization was a virtual lettre de cachet.[16]

The French newspapers did not restrict themselves to general charges; they also publicized specific cases of allegedly wrongful confinement. One such case was the Puyparlier affair. Upon the request of a Madame Puyparlier, the Charenton physician Rousselin examined the mental state of her husband in May 1869 and January 1870 in the company of Ludger Lunier, one of the inspectors-general of the national asylum system. Both times the two doctors found M. Puyparlier to be living alone in filth and in poor physical health. They concluded that he suffered from a "notable weakness" of his judgmental faculties and "moral sense," which led him to concoct extravagant schemes and left him vulnerable to financial swindlers. Yet these reasons in themselves were not enough to support the recommendation of the doctors that he be committed. Two other factors made the verdict of hospitalization seem more justifiable. First, Puyparlier had been a public nuisance in his hometown. He had several times been arraigned in court and fined for parading around town scantily clad and for urinating from his balcony onto the street below. Rousselin and Lunier lamented that the local magistrates had not had him committed as an involuntary patient, claiming that these acts of indecency represented threats to morality and public security. Second, although the doctors did not reveal whether Puyparlier's wife had requested it, they advised that because of his mental state he no longer be allowed to manage his own financial affairs. If it had been his wife's intention to strip him of his money and possessions, then he was clearly at a disadvantage when confronted by alienists acting in her interests. In short, Puyparlier's eccentric social behavior and his wife's probable inter-est in gaining control of his worldly goods made it more likely that Lunier and Rousselin would declare him a candidate for institution-alization.

Puyparlier's wife acted on the second medical certificate drawn up by Rousselin and Lunier, and in January 1870 he was sent to Charenton as a "voluntary" patient, his hospitalization having been requested by a family member. Almost immediately he began writ-ing to his lawyer and his friends, and only forty-eight hours after his arrival the newspapers published his complaints that he was the victim of a conspiracy to confine him in an insane asylum. Before being escorted to Charenton, Puyparlier had been allowed to eat lunch because of his undernourished state. He ate voraciously and consumed half a bottle of wine. He later fell asleep in the carriage and woke up in Charenton, claiming that his companions had given him a drug in his food to sedate him. When his story was publicized, there was a public outcry, and the minister of the interior author-ized Dr. Augustin Constans, Lunier's fellow inspector-general, to examine the patient. Constans confirmed the earlier diagnosis, as did a three-doctor commission. The commission agreed that de-spite Puyparlier's psychological condition he should be set free, although he would not be allowed to administer his own financial affairs. Nonetheless, Puyparlier was not freed, and another medical commission was called in to render its decision. On 19 February doctors Esprit Blanche, Auguste Motet, and Ambroise Tardieu in-terviewed Puyparlier and on 22 March announced that he was certi-fiably mad and should be hospitalized at Charenton.[17]

Another case that caught public attention involved a Mr. "C." of Rennes. The police apprehended him at four o'clock in the morning walking the streets dressed only in an overcoat, after having burnt his straw bed and his few possessions. A local doctor, asked to diagnose C.'s mental state, decided that C. had been a lunatic for a long time and periodically suffered from nervous states during which he became dangerous to social peace and public morality. By virtue of article 18 of the 1838 law, C. was involuntarily incarcerated in the public asylum of Saint-Méen. He was transferred to the public asylum of Quimper in November 1867. In September 1869 he wrote a letter to the commission considering changes to the 1838 law in which he complained of the brutality of the Saint-Méen asylum's ward assistants and of the punitive methods employed by the doctors of Rennes and Quimper to make their patients more manageable. He demanded damages for what he claimed was an illegal institutionalization. His charges were published in the *Electeur du Finistère* in November 1869.

The two alienists of the Rennes and Quimper asylums defended themselves in the *Annales médico-psychologiques* in January 1870. On his arrival at Saint-Méen, they claimed, C. was highly excited and grew violent, striking the hospital aides. A straightjacket was used to subdue him, but the two doctors maintained that he was not the victim of physical violence as he had reported. No signs of wounds could be detected, they declared. Furthermore, C. suffered from wild hallucinations that found expression in a series of letters he had written while hospitalized. They rested their defense on the threat C. posed to society and morality and on the intention of the 1838 law to safeguard law-abiding and sane citizens from dangerous lunatics. The managing editor of the *Electeur du Finistère* would not have been so ready to publish C.'s allegations, they argued, if he had custodial responsibility for someone like C., who paraded the streets naked or who might set his home on fire at any time.[18]

These accounts of alleged arbitrary hospitalization illustrate the ambiguities surrounding the role of the psychiatrist as stipulated by the 1838 law. While there were doubtlessly instances of dishonest asylum directors conspiring with certain families to put away unfortunate relatives, these were probably the exception rather than the rule. In the Puyparlier affair, for example, Rousselin proceeded cautiously by first assuring himself of Madame Puyparlier's good faith and then asking Lunier to join him to provide a second opinion. Physicians could also point out that in cases of involuntary confinement—the *placements d'office* that far outnumbered voluntary admissions—it was the civil authorities who initiated the admission proceedings and determined that someone constituted a danger to social peace. To focus on the medical role in the institutionalization process was to overlook the limited nature of the doctor's role in the majority of asylum admissions.

Alienists were in a difficult position. If a medical certificate of insanity endorsed hospitalization, they were vulnerable to the charge, however unfounded, of arbitrary confinement; if they pronounced someone sane and the individual committed a violent crime, the public could condemn them for being incompetent. Perhaps to reassure each other of their professional acumen, the editors of the *Annales médico-psychologiques* repeatedly published reports in the 1860s entitled "Lunatics at Liberty," which chronicled the gruesome crimes of ex-patients or escaped inmates. Psychiatrists plainly felt that if they were going to err, it was better that a person with marginally psychotic symptoms be hospitalized than set free and possibly commit a violent crime. Finally, it appears that the situation in France was basically the same as that in England in the mid-nineteenth century: psychiatrists were "the agents of a society determined to banish the mentally disturbed from its midst."[19] There was no finer expression of this social attitude than the 1838 law itself. The French public was acutely conscious of mental disease and worried, notably in the final third of the century, when social problems were often discussed in medical terms and metaphors, that lunatics posed a particularly serious threat to social order.[20] Psychiatrists had the thankless task of identifying and treating dangerous psychotics without infringing on the individual rights of French citizens.

But suspicions of wrongful confinement by psychiatrists were sometimes justified. Although alienists were not wholly responsible for incarcerating the insane, they still wielded considerable power in the form of the medical certificate necessary to ratify each admission to an asylum. From the two cases cited above, it is evident that the commitment process was based heavily on the potential danger to society presented by a nonhospitalized madman. Although doctors invariably stressed that hospitalization was for the lunatic's own good, they also underlined the importance to law and order of removing the insane from society. For example, Dr. Penquer, the president of the national association of French physicians, wrote to the *Electeur du Finistère* on 19 November 1869 reminding its readers that psychiatrists were devoted to treating "the saddest and the most dangerous of human infirmities." He maintained that criticism of mental medicine only served to discredit the asylum—"a useful institution that renders even more service to society than to the sick."[21]

Even in the "voluntary" admission of Puyparlier to Charenton, with its overtones of collusion between his wife and the medical consultants, standards of social behavior seem to have been a major consideration. Rousselin, Lunier, Constans, Blanche, Motet, and Tardieu all emphasized that Puyparlier's liberty compromised the security and property of other citizens. In a candid moment, Constans echoed Penquer's opinion of the asylum's usefulness: Puyparlier's place was in the asylum, "not that a cure is probable," he remarked, but because he could not be held responsible for his own affairs. In such a state of mind, Puyparlier was liable to commit "mad acts jeopardizing his health, his fortune, public morality, and even other people, for he could start a fire involuntarily."[22] Thus, accusations that psychiatrists exercised a subtle yet effective form of penal repression in helping to hospitalize individuals as dangers to society were not far from the truth. As C. himself alleged, an asylum was more a "house of correction" for enforcing behavioral conformity than a hospital for healing illness.[23] Some politicians agreed: the republican Léon Gambetta told the *Corps législatif* that the government's seeming indifference to the public pleas for restrictions on psychiatry proved that the interests of the imperial state and alienism were identical.[24]

The episode that probably drew the most attention to the relations between psychiatry and the French state was the Sandon affair. Léon Sandon was a lawyer who was confined in Charenton on the testimony of several Paris alienists. Because he had in his possession some incriminating letters from a Bonapartist cabinet minister, his confinement was cause for great suspicion. The liberal press protested loudly that Sandon was the victim of a government conspiracy perpetrated by psychiatric doctors. In 1865 Sandon prosecuted his own case in Paris, suing the alienists responsible for his internment. One of Sandon's accusations was that alienists were "police assassins" who out of self-interest were willing to follow orders and imprison enemies of the government.[25]

Alienists also tended to rely uncritically on conventional standards of sexual conduct in their diagnoses of insanity, thereby confusing madness with immorality and other varieties of nonconformity. Both Puyparlier and C. were supposedly guilty of public indecency, displaying in the process what alienists called a "lesion of the moral sense." That these actions brought them before the local magistrate was not particularly strange; that they were considered to be evidence of insanity indicates that alienists frequently served as guardians of respectability, morality, and the social system. Doctors' frequent lapses into this role—the result in large measure of their ignorance of the pathology of insanity—did not escape the notice of psychiatry's critics.

Because some alienists, such as Brierre de Boismont, made bold claims for psychiatry's medical authority, it was a particularly embarrassing blow to professional prestige when doctors could not agree whether to have a patient hospitalized. Compelled to defend their decisions on the basis of their experience in interpreting, identifying, and treating the symptoms of insanity, they could ill afford differences of opinions. For example, in February 1870 Puyparlier was examined by a commission of three physicians, whose conclusion that Puyparlier should be set free despite signs of "moral perversion" and mental weakness contradicted Rousselin's and Lunier's earlier conclusion. Although Henri Legrand du Saulle assured the readers of the *Gazette des hôpitaux* on 2 March 1870 that differences of opinion surfaced frequently in medical consultations, Lunier and Rousselin were worried that the publication of such disagreements would provoke grave misgivings about psychiatric acumen among laymen and "the portion of the medical public less familiar than we are" with mental pathology. These misgivings, they claimed, would strengthen suspicions that many inoffensive eccentrics were diagnosed as dangerous and eligible for committal and that psychiatrists had little regard for individual liberty. Psychiatric expertise was on trial; both Lunier and Rousselin believed that the major cause for concern in the Puyparlier affair was the prospect that the profession would lose credibility because not all the doctors involved favored Puyparlier's confinement.[26]

Probably the most persistent medical critic of alienism in the 1860s was Dr. Léopold Turck (1797–1887). Although not an alienist, Turck had firm opinions on the best way to treat the insane. For example, he advocated baths for mental patients for as long as forty-eight hours.[27] He also thought highly of "family treatment," a procedure followed at the Belgian lunatic colony of Gheel, which recommended boarding patients with local families.[28] Turck had only disdain for the insane asylum, where, he said, each year 3,000 inmates died because of cold, hunger, neglect, poor diet, despair, and strenuous labor. Asylums, he declared in a petition submitted to the Senate on 10 January 1865, turned acute cases of insanity into chronic cases and ended up killing rather than curing.[29]

Eugène Garsonnet, a secondary school teacher who was twice confined to Charenton, lent his voice to Turck's condemnation of French psychiatry. He wrote in 1867 that if it had not been for his social position he would have been committed for the rest of his life. He was shocked that psychological medicine had been authorized to enforce the 1838 law without proving first that it had developed a truly scientific understanding of the diseased mind.[30]

Many alienists were dismayed that other doctors were as suspicious as the public of psychiatry's expertise. In the Puyparlier affair the *Opinion médicale et scientifique* and *France médicale* published the accusations of the antipsychiatric spokesmen and, according to Lunier and Rousselin, did not hesitate to pass negative judgments on mental medicine.[31] The skepticism of physicians such as Turck, Castelnau, and Brunet made psychiatrists all the more conscious of their tenuous rapport with mainstream medicine and of their delicate social status.

The antipsychiatric campaign of the 1860s also exacerbated the troubled relations between alienists and the French magistracy. The Napoleonic Penal Code of 1810 had authorized judges to use discretion in determining the sanity of the accused and conceded that someone in a demented state could not be held responsible for criminal acts. An 1832 law gave judges and juries the right to mitigate the sentence specified in the 1810 code for a particular crime. However, neither the 1810 code nor the 1832 law specified which mental states could be considered extenuating, so judges increasingly relied on medical testimony in determining how responsible criminals were for their crimes. After 1838 a judge had the alternative of sending a criminal lunatic to an asylum rather than setting him or her free. Yet as alienists aggressively campaigned for recognition of their legal expertise, many magistrates and public prosecutors resented medical encroachment in their domain. By midcentury the legal profession had become highly skeptical of medical explanations of the mental state of criminals in cases in which the criminals exhibited no appreciable delirium or dementia. Alienists' disagreements about a criminal's responsibility gave psychiatry's enemies another issue to exploit.

One example of such exploitation was the Jeanson affair. On a night in late May 1868 a nineteen-year-old seminarian named Jeanson slit the throat of one of his fellow students and set fire to the seminary at Pont-à-Mousson. Jeanson was placed in the Maréville asylum on 2 June 1868, where at the request of the judge and public prosecutor he was examined by a group of doctors, including Henry Bonnet, the head physician at Maréville. Between June and the end of September Bonnet observed and talked with Jeanson and concluded that, despite the influence of a very strict education and the likelihood of a hereditary predisposition to insanity, Jeanson was not mad. Bonnet's testimony was crucial to the verdict of guilty with extenuating circumstances reached by the assize court at Nancy in February 1869. Jeanson was sentenced to twenty years hard labor.

This sentence was overturned in large part because of the intervention of B. A. Morel, who, after testifying in a widely publicized case in Germany, was in Nancy during the Jeanson trial. As the former medical director at Maréville, Morel was granted a short interview with the accused, whom he found to be suffering from an "instinctive or impulsive madness." Five doctors and Professor Behier, the inspector of private mental asylums in Paris, endorsed Morel's diagnosis. Morel then testified on behalf of the defense. Bonnet objected and wrote his account of the Jeanson affair for the May 1870 *Annales médico-psychologiques*. Morel answered him in the same volume, also entitling his article "The Truth of the Jeanson

Affair." Bonnet criticized Morel and his supporters for basing their opinions on a five-minute interview with the accused and on newspaper accounts of the trial.[32] Morel countered by accusing Bonnet of rendering testimony to satisfy public opinion, which Morel alleged favored a guilty verdict that would discredit the Catholic Church. In addition, he felt that Bonnet's animosity derived from an earlier episode in which Morel failed to acknowledge Bonnet's priority in a small matter of historical scholarship.[33] In any event, the dispute between Bonnet and Morel was typical of the acrimonious disagreements that plagued midcentury French mental medicine. Like the medical disputes in the well-publicized 1881–1882 trial of Charles Guiteau, the assassin of U.S. president James A. Garfield,[34] these were no credit to the alienist profession.

Perhaps because his diagnosis had been challenged originally, Bonnet stressed the professional consequences of the dispute. Bonnet insisted that magistrates and juries would cite this difference of opinion as evidence that alienists were incompetent and far too confident of their own expertise. He claimed that at least one judge had written to him that Bonnet's opponents had attributed three different mental illnesses to Jeanson. "This lad definitely is unduly rich in diseases," the magistrate had supposedly commented.[35]

Dr. H. Thulié, a former intern at Charenton, warned in an open letter to Dr. Auguste Motet in the *Annales médico-psychologiques* of the potential for psychiatric embarrassment. Thulié criticized the increasingly popular alienist concept of "reasoning mania," the mental state in which a pathological instinct was disguised by an apparently healthy mind, and charged that reliance on this diagnosis led to the confinement of eccentric but sane people. Psychiatric diagnostic expertise was even more dubious, he wrote, when episodes like the Jeanson affair were taken into consideration. The disagreement in the Jeanson case could not be dismissed easily, he added, because Bonnet was an ardent proponent of the 1838 law and an esteemed alienist, and therefore the doctors' failure to reach a consensus could not be attributed to any iconoclasm on Bonnet's part. If dissent was possible in the Jeanson affair—which involved some of the most illustrious French alienists of the day—then there was a good chance of error in any psychiatric diagnosis. The failure had more to do with the imprecision of alienist science than with the qualities of the doctors, Thulié insisted.[36]

Controversies such as these helped to sustain the mounting antipsychiatric sentiment of the 1860s, but what appeared to prod the imperial government to investigate the complaints against the psychiatric profession was the petition filed by Dr. Léopold Turck on 10 January 1865. A governmental report presented on 2 July 1867 conceded that the 1838 law's recommendation that judicial and administrative officials regularly visit the asylum was sometimes not observed and that a justice of the peace ought to verify each medical certificate authorizing institutionalization. The report nevertheless concluded that there was nothing fundamentally wrong with the law. Its spirit and intentions were above reproach, the report stated, and there were ample guarantees in its provisions against unjust asylum incarceration; psychiatry's enemies therefore had little reason to attack the 1838 law.[37]

However, the wave of complaints did not abate, and the government responded by conducting a survey of the departmental prefects' and alienists' opinions of the law. Of the one hundred and seventeen prefectural and seventy-seven medical responses received, the vast majority endorsed the law. Another commission was created in February 1869 to further study the 1838 law. It included members of the Senate and the *Corps législatif* as well as doctors Constans, Calmeil, and Tardieu. The secretary-general of the commission confirmed in a letter to the minister of the interior that since 1863 the asylum law had been the object of public attention. He also cited the earlier report and the minor changes made by the government in the original law. The new commission, he wrote, sought to improve the 1838 legislation even more in order to ensure individual liberty, although he and his colleagues agreed with the first commission that the criticisms contained in most petitions were unjust.[38]

Until 1870, then, psychiatry appeared for the most part to enjoy the support of the government and politicians against its treatment by the political press. Despite alienists' impression that the government had too readily bowed to public opinion by naming commissions of inquiry, medical powers had not been curtailed and the 1838 law had not been drastically changed.

However, on 21 March 1870 Léon Gambetta and Joseph Magnin, both members of the *Corps législatif*, introduced a bill that threatened to erode the administrative authority of psychiatry.[39]

Gambetta, who borrowed heavily from the arguments of Garsonnet and Turck, warned that anyone with a medical certificate could have another citizen committed as insane. What good could result from institutionalizing a mentally disturbed individual in a hospital whose environment was itself virtually pathogenic? he asked. The legislation of 1838, Gambetta claimed, had transformed what was essentially the "barbarous therapy" of incarceration into a sanctioned institution, thereby assuring that more would die than be cured by psychiatry.[40] Gambetta's and Magnin's bill stated that a medical certificate did not constitute sufficient proof that someone ought to be involuntarily hospitalized. It expressed Gambetta's distrust of "alienist science" and his refusal to attribute to psychiatry "an exclusive competence in the solution of the mysterious problems of the human mind."[41] Among its more significant proposals was the formation of a special jury, composed of a judge, notary, lawyer, justice of the peace, doctor, and a member of the local municipal council, to rule on each admission to and release from an asylum. The difference between this and earlier proposals was that it would not simply reinforce juridical authority in the hospitalization process but would also reduce the role of the doctor. Gambetta's bill, "one of the most audacious" attempts to reform the 1838 law and weaken medical authority,[42] was particularly galling to psychiatrists because it transferred some of their power to the legal profession.

Gambetta's and Magnin's bill failed to receive a serious hearing. A bill based on the studies of yet another commission and of the Société de législation comparée met the same fate in 1872. The issue did not disappear, however. In 1881 a new commission was formed; it presented a bill that was introduced to the Senate on 25 November 1882 by Senator Théophile Roussel, a member of the Société médico-psychologique, who filed a lengthy report on the bill with the Senate on 20 May 1884.[43] Roussel's report called for greater judicial involvement in commitment and release procedures, the creation of special quarters for epileptics and the mentally retarded, the elimination of private asylums, the establishment of provisional asylums in which suspected lunatics could be observed before confinement in regular asylums, and the retention of clerical asylums.[44] Roussel's bill was passed by the Senate on 11 March 1887 with many of its recommendations either eliminated or modified, but it failed to reach the floor of the Chamber of Deputies. On 3 December 1890 Joseph Reinach resurrected it in the Chamber. This latest bill also revived the antialienist sentiments of the Gambetta bill. Reinach denied that psychiatry was based on a science that justified its role in the internment of lunatics and dismissed the notion that the collective hospitalization of the insane in an asylum was a salutary measure. The insane asylum was little more than a prison, according to Reinach.[45] His bill also did not receive a reading in the Chamber, yet he and a fellow deputy produced in 1893 another bill critical of alienism calling for the usual reforms: the creation of special asylums for the mentally retarded, quarters for provisional observation, the elimination of private asylums, and the increased surveillance of all asylums by nonmedical officials. This bill also failed.

The bill that came closest to success was introduced by Deputy Fernand Dubief, former medical director of the Marseille asylum, and debated in early 1907.[46] Dubief's bill tried to break the medical monopoly on the internment and release of the insane, but Dubief was careful to praise the medical profession frequently and to describe the alienist as the key to a more just system of treatment and social defence. On the whole, alienists were not unhappy with the bill and welcomed the introduction of special quarters for alcoholics and the mentally retarded. They also applauded the expanded role for medical experts in the management of the many varieties of social deviance foreseen by the Dubief bill. They felt that the progress of mental medicine was closely tied to their future function as auxiliary "police of moral discipline," especially with regard to the social problem of alcoholism and its influence on crime.[47] Unfortunately for psychiatry, the Dubief bill languished in the Senate after passing in the Chamber.

The acceptance by most psychiatrists of the Dubief bill indicated that the atmosphere surrounding the discussion and reform of the 1838 law was less charged with distrust and enmity around 1900 than it had been just before the Franco-Prussian war. As acceptance of psychiatry slowly grew in the late nineteenth century, alienists increasingly felt little need to act defensively. They also grew less militant about the usefulness of the asylum as they began to question whether their social role ought to be restricted to institutional practice. While public indignation could still be aroused in 1907 over allegations of arbitrary confinement, less credence was given to the allegations than in previous decades. Antipsychiatric sentiment after the fall of the Second Empire in 1870 and the founding of the Third Republic (1870–1940) was never as sustained as it was in the 1860s.

This did not mean that after 1870 press attacks on alienism disappeared. They continued throughout the 1870s and 1880s, buoyed by the published criticisms of leading legal experts.[48] Public suspicion of psychiatry was intense shortly after the Franco-Prussian War. For example, the alienists Prosper Lucas and Valentin Magnan and two other doctors from the Sainte-Anne asylum offered a series of public clinical lectures on mental illness, but shortly after the series began on 9 March 1873, the protests of the Paris newspapers forced the prefect of the Seine to halt the lectures on the grounds that exhibiting the insane created a scandal and divulged professional secrets. Despite drawing a large audience for the inaugural lecture, the series did not reopen for another three years and then only after a strongly worded protest by the Société médico-psychologique directed to the minister of public instruction and the ministry of the interior.[49]

There were other indications that the public held alienists in low regard in the early years of the Third Republic. In 1872 the Paris public flocked to the Odéon theater to see a play entitled *The Baroness*. In this drama a calculating young woman married an elderly and wealthy count, whom she was assured had only six months to live. When she and her lover, a Dr. Yarley, were discovered in each other's arms, her husband flew into a rage. Acting quickly and with the complicity of her lover, she had her husband confined to a mental hospital. Dr. Yarley had a crisis of conscience and released the husband, who promptly went home and strangled his wife. After being arrested, he proclaimed himself insane and hence irresponsible for his actions.[50]

The box office success of *The Baroness* and the press attacks of the next two decades show that the antipsychiatric movement of the 1860s was not a fleeting phenomenon. Between 1860 and the turn of the century the French public believed that psychiatry constituted a dangerously repressive force and that medical expertise in the care of the mad was a fraud.[51] The continued unpopularity of psychiatry also demonstrated that its alliance with the Bonapartist regime—forged with difficulty in the 1860s—had helped to stigmatize its practitioners during the first three decades of the Third Republic. Despite its liberal and republican origins, alienism in the 1860s had been attacked as energetically by the anti-Bonapartist left as by the clerical and conservative right.

Rather than ignoring the attacks of their critics, alienists in the 1860s reacted defensively when confronted with this pervasive public suspicion. Their concern with lay hostility can be measured by the Société médico-psychologique's debates in the 1860s, in which psychiatrists stressed that the insane were a threat to society and that madness could be effectively treated only in a mental hospital.

At issue during the antipsychiatric controversy was the 1838 law and its recommended form of public assistance to the insane, the asylum. The asylum's social, economic, and medical usefulness became the main topic of discussion at the Société médico-psychologique between October 1864 and February 1866. Jules Falret opened the discussions by proposing that the Société consider the merits of four alternative means of public assistance: first, sending inoffensive and incurable lunatics back to their families; second, housing the insane with the inhabitants in the neighborhood of the asylum—what the English called the "cottage system"; third, the creation of entire villages for the mad, such as the Gheel colony in Belgium; and fourth, the establishment of agricultural farms affiliated with a mental hospital. Yet what followed was no dispassionate, disinterested, or empirical examination of different ways of caring for the mad, for the Société's alienists repeatedly expressed their belief that psychiatry's claim to specialized knowledge of insanity and its status as a legitimate corps of professional functionaries were threatened when the usefulness of the asylum was debated. For example, Dr. A. Linas observed that the discussions at the Société dealt with "the very future" of psychiatry.[52] Dr. J. B. Parchappe maintained that the debates were addressed to the popular attack on psychological medicine, a movement that demanded the destruction of psychiatry and denigrated asylums and the medical officials who staffed them.[53] For Jules Falret as well, the antipsychiatric movement was "a veritable crusade" to scrap the principles that had guided mental medicine and asylum administration since the beginning of the century.[54] A disquieting opinion came from Dr. Jaromir Mundy, an asylum doctor from Germany, who, when introduced to the Société as a member on 26 December 1864, declared that a radical reform of the asylum system was an urgent necessity.[55] The minutes of the Société's meetings between 1864 and 1866 reveal that almost every alienist disagreed with Mundy and thought that the existing public asylum was the best means for treating all forms of mental derangement.

The years of attacks on psychiatry had left alienists confused and unsure of the best way to respond publicly. On 14 November 1864 Dr. Achille Foville suggested that the Société issue a brochure containing the minutes of its discussions of the national asylum system. Foville hoped that the brochure would serve as a statement of alienist confidence in the 1838 law and consequently convince the public that psychiatry was performing a rigorously scientific duty rather than a conspiratorial task. He advised sending it to administrative officials in the national government, who, impressed by the collective declaration of psychiatrists, would endorse the specialist "mission" of mental medicine.[56] Not all the Société's members agreed with Foville. Alfred Maury and Dr. Legrand du Saulle opposed any official attempt to disprove the allegations of the press, which they feared could be seen as meddling in political affairs and could result in an imperial reprimand of the Société and censorship of the *Annales médico-psychologiques*. Alienists were caught between society and the government. By actively opposing the popular forces that cried for its dissolution, psychiatry ran the risk of alarming the Napoleonic authorities. By staying within the domain of medical science, they left themselves vulnerable to the charges of the reformers, charges that the state seemed to take seriously.

The same held true for the issue of the dangerousness of the mad, debated at the Société médico-psychologique between July 1868 and July 1869. The issue was particularly troublesome for alienists. It was tied, Jules Falret reminded the Société, to the recent discussions of the 1838 law and psychiatry in the newspapers, courts, legislative assemblies, and executive councils of government. Psychiatry's critics had contended that a lunatic should be hospitalized involuntarily only if a crime had been committed. However, in many of the involuntary *placements d'office* there had been no crime committed. According to Falret, the public was wrong to blame the alienist for this situation because in virtually every hospitalization the commitment proceedings had been initiated by the family of the patient or the authorities, who in their eagerness to institutionalize the patient exaggerated the potential for suicide or other forms of violence. Falret conceded that among these many admissions there were some inoffensive lunatics, but he nonetheless believed that the system authorized by the 1838 law was still the soundest. Because many of the insane were potentially dangerous, he and most of his colleagues considered it wiser to institutionalize the vast majority of the insane while endeavoring to formulate precise criteria with which to distinguish between harmless and dangerous lunatics.[57]

Concern about the potential for violence also influenced the decision of psychiatrists to discharge patients. The enemies of psychiatry claimed that alienists exaggerated the dangerousness of their hospitalized patients as a way of postponing their release. This especially applied to involuntary patients whose mental state compromised public order and the safety of other citizens. Doctors were worried that the premature release of a patient could lead to criminal violence and therefore to charges of psychiatric incompetence.[58] Dr. Ludger Lunier acknowledged that even the most experienced alienist disliked formulating a categorical diagnosis in these cases. Speaking to the Société médico-psychologique, Lunier argued that some cases of madness were clear cut, but he reminded his listeners never to overlook the possible "terrible consequences" of releasing a patient before there was a cure. Confronted with a debatable case of lunacy, Lunier reasoned that the alienist did best when he authorized isolation in an insane asylum, thereby avoiding a possibly scandalous situation for mental medicine.[59]

Lunier's speech suggests that public spokesmen were justified in accusing alienists of functioning as police when they diagnosed the potential for violence of certain lunatics. While insisting that the distinction between dangerous and harmless lunatics was valid and that psychiatrists were best able to make this distinction, alienists agreed that "in principle, all madmen were dangerous," as Lunier asserted,[60] and ought to be hospitalized. Some alienists, like Falret, Henri Dagonet, and Eugène Billod, admitted that they viewed almost every lunatic as dangerous, an opinion that bothered Dr. H. Belloc, the medical director of the asylum at Alençon (Orne). Speaking to the Société on 14 December 1868, Belloc traced psychiatry's tendency to consider all patients as dangerous to the med-

ical inability to produce a scientific definition of the dangerous lunatic. Antipsychiatric spokesmen had exploited this gap in alienist
knowledge, Belloc said, in order to demonstrate that doctors had
little justification for being involved in what was properly an administrative—not an etiological, diagnostic, or therapeutic—problem.
As an asylum alienist himself, Belloc was no opponent of mental
medicine, but he felt that it was vitally important for alienists to
recognize that the public slander of them stemmed from their diagnostic and therapeutic shortcomings.[61] If Belloc was more candid
than his colleagues about the inability of alienists to define each
patient's potential for violence, he was no less anxious to end the
public criticism of asylum medicine. He simply thought that the
problem could not be solved if psychiatrists refused to believe that
they were in any way responsible for it.

The principal effect of the strident public criticism of mental
medicine was to convince alienists that as representatives of medical science they were isolated and at the mercy of popular movements. They viewed themselves as threatened by irrational cultural
forces that ignored their humanitarian achievements and scientific
progress and that sought to dismantle the asylum system. They also
began to see themselves as deserted by their earlier political allies,
the liberals. As this sense of social isolation deepened in the final
third of the century, alienists increasingly identified their interests
with those of the state in order to make themselves less vulnerable
to popular attacks. The gradual reinforcement of this mentality encouraged alienists to believe that opposition to asylum medicine
was the same as opposition to constituted political authority.

A favorite tactic of psychiatrists like Parchappe, Motet, Morel,
and Ernest Mesnet was to accuse those who called for the liberation
of the insane of insanity themselves, so convinced were they that
the modern asylum was testimony to progress and to the benevolence of their profession.[62] Others, like Foville and Dagonet, saw
the Catholic Church behind the demands of the political press to
place the insane beyond the reach of medicine.[63] At issue for alienists concerned with professional prerogatives was, as Parchappe put
it, "the authority legally acquired by the medical corps" since the
beginning of the century.[64] As Falret told the Société médico-psychologique on 27 July 1868, it was urgent that alienists formulate
precise criteria for diagnosing dangerousness in their patients; if

they did not, other professional groups would do so, thereby eliminating medical competition and clinical experience from an area of
social practice that rightly belonged to alienism.[65] To the average
alienist the science of psychiatry represented sixty years of experience living with and treating the mad. Now psychiatry's enemies
were claiming that all this experience had merely produced prejudice and a dangerously conventional attitude toward those who
exhibited disordered thinking. Brierre de Boismont probably
summed up the feelings of many alienists when he told the Société
that he found the accusations of wrongful confinement to be "pro-
foundly distressing" and confessed that, were he not absolutely convinced that the accusations were false, he would regret ever having
taken up a career as an alienist.[66]

As the malaise among alienists continued into the 1870s and
1880s, a growing number of psychiatrists agreed that scientific values and popular tastes were inimical. According to Henry Bonnet,
commenting on the way in which the drama *The Baroness* reflected
the common sentiments of the times, the public was poorly educated and therefore highly susceptible to malicious and sensation-
alist propaganda spread by those who had no respect for science
or "social institutions." Bonnet viewed alienism as a defender of
science, whose interests he in turn equated with those of social
order. Consequently, Bonnet and other alienists believed, psychiatry was bound to suffer when scientific authority was undermined
by populist forces.[67]

Fifteen years later, alienists still felt that the antagonism between medical science and the popular *mentalité* was strong. Ben-
jamin Ball, the first to hold the chair of mental pathology at the Paris
Faculty of Medicine, recounted on 16 August 1887 the circumstances surrounding the Sellière affair. A doctor from the Prefecture of Police in Paris had authorized the release of a Baron
Sellière from Jules Falret's asylum. After he left the hospital, the
press published his account of his confinement. He alleged that his
medical custodians had given him hypodermic injections to disori-
ent his thinking, had tried to asphyxiate him, and had forced him to
drink a corrosive liquid while he was restrained in a straightjacket.
Ball protested in Falret's defense for, he said, as a faculté professor
he had less to fear than a public asylum doctor by speaking out on
the issue. He declared that "contemporary morals" made it virtually

impossible for "men of science" to receive a fair hearing. The press, Ball claimed, preferred to publish outrageous accounts like Sellière's rather than the soberly scientific diagnoses of trained physicians; and this especially held true, Ball added, for those doctors who "have the misfortune to attend to the insane."[68]

French alienism entered the final third of the century suffering from what might be termed a state-of-siege mentality. Beginning in the 1860s their competence and intentions as asylum physicians had been seriously questioned by other corporate groups such as the legal profession that sought to undermine their prerogatives and by political elements that were eager to find a scapegoat on whom to vent their anti-Bonapartist rancor. But even some doctors recognized that there was some substance to the antipsychiatric charges, for alienists had shown themselves to be willing to perform police functions in the service of the imperial state. The awareness of this compounded the already visceral sense of isolation and uneasiness that had characterized mental medicine since the early 1800s. Psychiatrists could refer to no authoritative or professionally approved model of pathology that, by making sense of their clinical data in psychological, biological, and social terms, could forestall allegations of ignorance, incompetence, and cognitive confusion. Without such a model, antipsychiatric attitudes were likely to harden, and the troubles of alienism were likely to continue.

Chapter Six

Hereditarianism, the Clinic, and Psychiatric Practice in Nineteenth-Century France

By the early years of the Third Republic the psychiatric profession in France had reason to feel anxious and defensive about its social status. Antipsychiatric sentiment was running high, fanned by journalistic allegations of wrongful confinement and medical ignorance and incompetence. Public outrage had called into question the existence of the asylum, the social usefulness of the 1838 law, and the integrity, expertise, and authority of psychiatry. Furthermore, the profession had been stigmatized as Bonapartist because its efforts to appear conciliatory to the imperial state had not escaped the attention of ardent republicans like Gambetta. Under the pressure of trying to adapt to the shifting cultural climate between 1848 and 1900, alienists began to develop hereditarian approaches to mental disease as a way of legitimizing their participation in the moral treatment of madness, their role as purveyors of essential medical information, and the existence of the insane asylum. The popularity of hereditarianism grew until the turn of the century as alienists depicted themselves as humanitarian, positivist, and biomedically erudite asylum doctors committed to political order and scientific progress.

The Rise of Hereditarianism within French Psychiatry in the Second Half of the Nineteenth Century

Psychiatric references to the influence of heredity on mental disease, although not unprecedented,[1] multiplied dramatically in the second half of the nineteenth century. Jacques Moreau de Tours wrote prolifically about the biological effects of heredity on mental and nervous diseases. Other alienists contributed to the vogue of hereditarianism after midcentury. In the first volume of his *Philosophical and Physiological Treatise on Natural Heredity*,[2] the psychiatrist Prosper Lucas wrote that in his day heredity was "an obscure and great problem," but the time was ripe to finally achieve a "rational understanding" of the issue. To accommodate those who stressed the similarities between parents and offspring and those who paid more attention to the dissimilarities, Lucas proposed that there were two broad biological laws governing the evolution of a species: a "law of heredity" that operated to perpetuate physical and moral characteristics; and a "law of *innéité*," which represented the capacity of nature to spontaneously produce variations among members of the same species.[3] In the years following the appearance of his book, alienists and other writers tended to reject Lucas's second law.[4] But whatever the scientific value and popularity of his laws, Lucas's detailed study of heredity indicated that morbid heredity was beginning to interest alienists in a significant way.

One psychiatrist who followed Lucas's lead was his colleague at the Société médico-psychologique, Ulysée Trélat. In 1856 Trélat contended that psychiatry had been preoccupied for too long with the external causes of insanity, a situation that engendered confusion regarding its etiology. He recommended that physicians dramatically change their way of viewing the issue and recognize the importance of heredity, the great "internal" cause. He conceded that heredity was not a new issue, but he believed that it was much more important than had been recognized previously.[5] The alienist Emile Renaudin agreed. Never before had the appreciation of heredity's role in mental pathogenesis been so widespread, in part, he argued, because heredity seemed to accumulate the acquired pathological characteristics of each generation, producing the high incidence of disease evident in midcentury France. He cited alco-

holism, which apparently occurred in epidemic proportions during
the Second Empire, as one of the acquired characteristics that contributed to the growing wave of hereditary disease.[6]

With the possible exception of Moreau, the most important
alienist writer on hereditarianism in the 1850s was Bénédict-
Augustin Morel (1809–1873). Born in Vienna, the son of a supplier
to the Napoleonic armies, Morel was left by his father in the hands
of the clergy in 1814. He entered a seminary as an adolescent and
remained a devout Catholic all his life, although he never joined the
priesthood. He lived in Paris as a journalist and medical.student
from 1831 to 1839, when he took up the study of mental pathology.
While pursuing his medical studies, he lived in poverty, sharing
accommodations with the physiologist Claude Bernard, who introduced him to the Salpêtrière alienist J. P. Falret. Falret's influence proved decisive in attracting Morel to mental medicine.
During the 1840s Morel contributed to the *Annales médico-psychologiques*, traveled around Europe inspecting the different
forms of medical assistance to the insane, and was part of Philippe
Buchez's social circle. In 1848 Morel accepted an asylum appointment at Maréville, where he stayed until 1856. From 1856 to the
end of his life Morel served as medical director of the St. Yon asylum at Rouen. He died there of diabetes in 1873.[7]

In 1857 Morel published the major work of his career, *Treatise
on the Intellectual, Moral, and Physical Degeneracy of the Human
Race*. According to him, factors such as alcoholism, immorality,
poor diet, and unhealthy domestic and occupational conditions produced a pathological sequence that characterized the lineage of
some families. Members of these families exhibited the symptoms
of neurosis, mental alienation, imbecility, idiocy, and sterility over
the course of four generations. Morel based his theory on his observations of working-class communities in Rouen and families in
isolated rural areas. The degenerative mental and physical characteristics of these families constituted a deviation from the "primitive
type" of the human species, a type Morel equated with the biblical
Adam. The key element in the degenerative process was heredity.
Like Renaudin and Trélat, Morel believed that the time had come
to expand the meaning of heredity.[8] He argued that heredity transmitted an organic disposition to not only a particular disease but
also a flawed condition of the nervous system—nervous "di-

athesis"—that could produce a variety of neurological and psychical disturbances.[9] As Buchez reminded the Société médico-psychologique in 1857, Morel's conception of heredity had serious implications for the entire human race, since heredity was viewed conventionally as a simple predisposition that affected the health of only the individual patient.[10]

Morel's studies of degeneracy led him to an equally innovative classification of mental diseases. In 1860 Morel proposed that alienists discard the customary method of classification, associated with Pinel and Esquirol, which identified the varieties of insanity according to psychological symptoms recorded at the moment a patient was admitted to an asylum. Morel recommended instead a method of classification based on etiology or causes. Because he believed heredity accounted for many different mental symptoms, he argued that the diseases they conventionally represented ought to be combined in one nosological category called *hereditary madness*. After acknowledging Moreau's endorsement of this concept in his 1859 *Morbid Psychology*, Morel told the Société médico-psychologique that he counted on "time" and his younger colleagues to justify his hypothesis of a distinct class of "hereditary madmen" comprising those who combined apparent reason with behavioral deviance and those who were severely retarded.[11]

Alienist interest in morbid heredity increased in the 1860s as more psychiatrists grew critical of the traditional classification of mental diseases. For example, Dr. G. Doutrebente, one of Morel's student interns, won the 1868 *Prix Esquirol* awarded by the Société médico-psychologique for his treatment of the question of hereditary madness. His goal, like Morel's, was to establish the physical, affective, and intellectual signs that indicated hereditary madness. This was an important consideration because some psychiatrists, while rejecting the old classification scheme of Pinel and Esquirol, also criticized Morel's etiologically-oriented method of classification for failing to specify the characteristics that identified a hereditary psychological disorder. According to Doutrebente, such characteristics did exist and included bilateral flattening of the cranium, receding forehead, undersized genitalia, compulsion to suicide and murder, obsessional ideas, and erratic behavior since childhood. The diagnostic and prognostic task was much simpler, he claimed, when the alienist focused on these symptoms.[12]

Another indication of increased alienist interest in hereditarianism was the series of discussions at the Société médico-psychologique of the role of pathological inheritance in the etiology of mental alienation. The meetings began on 30 December 1867 with the admission that medicine lacked precise information on the proportion of children who became ill in families stigmatized by hereditary predisposition. As Jules Baillarger conceded, it was "an extremely grave question" because doctors were often asked by patients and their families if the presence of morbid heredity was fatal or ruled out marriage. In order to discover the relevant facts, Charles Lasègue proposed restricting the discussion to the question of the hereditary influence of epilepsy. He believed that in view of the inexact medical and popular theories of heredity, it was prudent to begin its study with a limited goal. His friend Morel was bolder and urged the Société to discuss the physical and psychological characteristics that he claimed identified hereditary insanity.[13]

During these discussion in early 1868, it became apparent that the members of the society were divided in their opinions regarding heredity. One group, headed by Louis Delasiauve, admitted only that epilepsy could be directly inherited from epileptic parents; that is, they believed that heredity passed on only specific diseases to progeny. The other group followed Morel's and Moreau's lead and argued that epilepsy was tied through heredity to other nervous disorders and diseases such as hysteria, alcoholism, scrofula, tuberculosis, and rickets. They believed that in some families heredity transmitted a diathesis, an organic condition that tended to make nerve tissue respond to stimuli pathologically. A diathesis was a constitutional and inherited disposition to disease, which from the medical standpoint was more important than any specific disease. As an example of this condition, Dr. Auguste Voisin cited the case of an epileptic patient who had two maternal uncles who died of tuberculosis, a tubercular and epileptic mother, a retarded brother, a scrofulous sister, and four other siblings who died of meningitis, croup, typhoid fever, and congenital phimosis.[14]

From the 1860s to the 1880s, hereditarianism continued to gain popularity within mental medicine. While some alienists refused even by the turn of the century to accept the theory of hereditary diathesis, they were far outnumbered by psychiatrists who wrote extensively on heredity and the affective and behavioral characteristics of degenerates and hereditary lunatics. Hereditarianism appeared to gain acceptance particularly among the young generation of psychiatrists who began their internships in the 1860s, although it also gained some converts from previous generations, including the prominent Alexandre Brierre de Boismont. In 1851 Brierre de Boismont had complained that Moreau's hereditarian theories were tainted with materialism,[15] but by the mid-1870s he had become an unabashed proponent of hereditarianism. When Morel died in 1873, Brierre de Boismont praised his theory of degeneracy and his recognition of the pathological impact of heredity on successive generations.[16] In 1875 he applauded Théodule Ribot's *Heredity: A Psychological Study of its Phenomena, Laws, Causes, and Consequences* for its treatment of the hereditary issue and reliance on alienist authors such as Morel and Moreau. He also reversed his earlier position and endorsed Ribot's conclusion that the inheritance of psychological traits was a biophysiological fact of heredity.[17] In short, Brierre de Boismont, one of the most psychologically oriented alienists of the nineteenth century, had done a complete about-face since the 1850s.

The 1880s marked the heyday of hereditarianism in French psychiatry. One of the people most responsible for hereditarianism's success was Valentin Magnan of the Sainte-Anne asylum, "the most illustrious representative of French psychiatry at the end of the nineteenth century."[18] Magnan was born 16 March 1835 and began his medical studies at the university in Montpellier. By 1863 he was in Paris competing for an internship. He worked at Bicêtre and Salpêtrière for two years and defended his medical thesis in 1866. The next year he was appointed head physician of the *bureau des admissions* at the newly built Sainte-Anne mental hospital, which he left in 1912, four years before his death.

Before the early 1880s Magnan's work had been devoted chiefly to experimental research on the organic lesions of the brain and the pathophysiological effects of alcoholic intoxication. Between 1881 and 1897 he concentrated on the analysis of the protean mental states of Morel's hereditary degenerates.[19] Magnan believed that Morel had sufficiently demonstrated the physical signs of hereditary madness and that the affective and intellectual signs of hereditary insanity were what needed to be identified.[20]

Magnan's efforts to make this identification led to the seminal debates at the Société médico-psychologique between March 1885 and July 1886 on the physical, moral, and intellectual signs of hereditary insanity. These debates marked the rise of hereditarianism in psychiatry in the 1880s because the choice of topic indicates that hereditarianism had become an acceptable etiological and nosological position.

During the 1885–1886 discussions, Jules Falret, who in the 1860s had opposed Morel's etiological classification of mental illnesses based on heredity, swung over to Magnan's side, as did many other alienists. Dr. Jules Christian, one of Magnan's opponents, conceded in May 1886 that "with the ideas that reign in pathology today," doctors were led to cite heredity as "the almost sole efficient cause of mental alienation."[21] Magnan also believed that there was more consensus than disagreement on the hereditary issue. Most psychiatrists, he told the Société, accepted the clinical reality of a class of patients united on the basis of similar hereditary conditions. Consequently, Magnan and Falret could argue over what mental and nervous illnesses ought to be included in Morel's class of *héréditaires,* while still agreeing that hereditary insanity was a clinically valuable nosological category. Similarly, while some doctors continued to believe that it was wrong to postulate the existence of a neuropathic diathesis transmitted by heredity, the majority of alienists agreed that heredity endowed a large number of patients with a host of physical and mental problems. If psychiatrists were sometimes unable to identify these problems exactly, they were nonetheless convinced that they existed and were due to morbid hereditary predisposition.[22]

The pervasiveness of hereditarianism in mental medicine in the 1880s was further indicated by the emergence of the theory of the "neuropathic family." This theory was proposed by Dr. Charles Féré in 1884. Féré, a neuropsychiatrist and member of the Salpêtrière school headed by J. M. Charcot, hypothesized the existence of a family of neurological and psychical diseases that could all be traced to the same hereditary lesion. He repeated and expanded the notion of a hereditary neuropathic diathesis by attributing to heredity a host of congenital deformities and neurological syndromes, such as chorea and locomotor ataxia, that had been recently described by Charcot and his followers in neuroanatomy. He linked these disorders to the various forms of mental alienation and to the diseases that were customarily believed to be hereditary in origin.[23] In essence Féré completed Moreau's project of the 1850s and 1860s to determine which chronic diseases could be associated with insanity on the basis of morbid heredity.

The appearance of Féré's theory of a neuropathic family, the endeavors of Magnan to confirm Morel's theory of hereditary degeneracy, and the debates at the Société médico-psychologique all signal hereditarianism's dominance in psychiatric thinking at the end of the nineteenth century. Alienists tended to focus on the role of heredity in mental pathogenesis to the exclusion of other factors, such as occupational stress, as one psychiatrist complained in 1883.[24] Indeed, by the 1880s few doctors believed mental and nervous diseases could be acquired. The neuropsychiatrist Jules Dejerine even predicted in 1886 that "acquired nervous affections" would dwindle substantially in number in the future, overshadowed by the symptomatological changes that hereditary diatheses would undergo as they were passed from one generation to the next.[25]

Hereditarian alienists were undeterred when a lunatic's family history showed little evidence of certifiable mental pathology. As Féré noted, heredity often "accumulated" over several generations before it manifested itself in a virulent form. For hereditary "taint" to be deduced, it was enough that a patient's ancestors had been "inventive" or eccentric, that they were "enthusiasts" or "spendthrifts," or simply that they had exhibited mildly neurotic behavior.[26] When Doutrebente was faced with a case of pronounced madness without evidence of bad heredity, for example, he refused to accept that the illness had no hereditary origins and solved the apparent puzzle by assuming that the patient was the result of an adulterous liaison.[27]

Despite this alienist taste for hereditary explanation, critics within psychiatry itself pointed out the anomalies of hereditarianism. For example, Dr. Bouchereau of the Société médico-psychologique criticized Magnan for blurring the distinction between those who acquired their mental illness and those who inherited it. Bouchereau asked how Magnan could assume that the unhealthy offspring of alcoholic parents always inherited their mental malady. The child of an alcoholic mother, he claimed, could be severely traumatized by accidents or physical abuse, or alcohol could be introduced into the blood of the infant through its mother's milk.

These influences or the exposure of the fetus to other disorders could contribute to disease in the next generation. Why should heredity be viewed as paramount in importance? Bouchereau asked.[28] He and Dr. Jules Christian accused Magnan of ignoring the environmental and traumatic elements that contributed to mental pathogenesis.[29]

Hereditarianism was beset with other difficulties. As late as 1886 it had to be admitted that statistical studies had divulged little reliable information on the incidence of hereditary insanity.[30] Christian was correct that alienists had little knowledge of heredity's laws. "What we possess today is the intuition of heredity's laws much more than the laws themselves," he said, and he openly questioned whether "an element so imperfectly understood, so capricious in its appearances, can in sound logic serve as the basis for an entire doctrine."[31] It was also conceded that in the majority of cases of hereditary madness there was no observable and characteristic somatic lesion, as there was for severely retarded patients. Magnan could only postulate that hereditary insanity was due to diffuse functional changes in the cellular tissue of the cerebrospinal system.[32] And whereas early champions of hereditarianism, like Morel and Buchez, had argued that a clinical approach based on the existence of a class of hereditary patients improved the chances for accurate prognosis, Louis Delasiauve claimed that because the physiological effect of the "predisposing germ" of heredity was unknown, an alienist could not say with certainty whether someone with a hereditary taint would fall ill.[33] Some French psychiatrists did not even use the diagnostic category of hereditary insanity. For instance, in his statistical account of admissions to Paris asylums processed through the Special Infirmary at the Prefecture of Police between 1872 and 1885, Dr. Augustin Planès expressed his surprise that none of the medical certificates endorsing hospitalization indicated the diagnosis of hereditary madness or degeneracy, a curious phenomenon given that two of the three doctors who issued these certificates were Lasègue and Henri Legrand du Saulle, both proponents of hereditarianism.[34]

Faced with the patent weaknesses and inconsistencies of hereditarian explanations of psychopathology, alienists were compelled to adopt an extremely flexible and inexact interpretation of hereditary madness. According to Dr. Paul Garnier, the confusion over whether heredity signified the inheritance of innate or acquired characteristics meant that hereditary madness took on an equivocal meaning for alienists, a reproach he thought justified when referring to similarly labile medical terms that enjoyed great popularity.[35] Indeed, this confusion surrounding hereditarianism as a medical concept may instead have been an important source of its popularity. To understand why this was so it is necessary to examine how French physicians used hereditarian explanations in the last half of the nineteenth century.

Hereditarianism and Psychiatric Practice

Alienists' loose reliance on hereditarianism suggests that they consciously or unconsciously capitalized on its imprecision in order to divert attention from their ignorance of what caused mental illness. Appeals to the hegemony of heredity in pathology "were a substitute by default for an unknown causality . . . , expressing at once the dream and the illusion of a mastery of the phenomena."[36] The "criteria of heredity" that doctors applied in clinical psychiatry were "extremely diffuse" and so "permitted of many different interpretations in accordance with each researcher's special orientation."[37] Because hereditarian accounts by alienists were ultimately so vague, the substantial gaps in psychiatric knowledge could be disguised and the illusion of consensus could be sustained despite the customary professional disagreements.

The usefulness of a broadly defined hereditarianism did not stop there, however. The use—and abuse—of hereditarianism discloses that alienists also borrowed Morel's terms because they enabled psychiatrists to include under the category of "patient" a substantial number of people who behaved and thought erratically yet were rarely believed to be mad. As Morel described them in 1860, they were "hereditarily afflicted individuals who live their whole life in an intellectually abnormal state, who periodically commit eccentric and dissolute acts, whose minds are, so to speak, in a permanent state of wandering without ever succumbing to dementia or paralysis."[38] These individuals were precisely those "lucid *aliénés*" whom Ulysée Trélat described in 1861. Found outside as often as inside the asylum, these people upset the order of everyday life with their alcoholism, kleptomania, sexual perversions, suicidal tendencies, defiance of constituted authority, and sporadic violence.[39] By classifying them as sufferers of hereditary insanity, alienists could argue that these persons were susceptible to sinister, irresistible impulses caused by a damaged nervous system, thereby strengthening physicians' reputation for expertise in criminal law and alienists' reputation as specialized diagnosticians.

The difficulty for alienists was that many disturbed individuals whom doctors were inclined to certify as insane had prolonged periods of lucidity and rational thinking. What led alienists to diagnose them as insane was their ostensible inability to use reason and willpower to prevent themselves from behaving immorally and criminally. Psychiatrists variously described these persons as suffering from "lucid madness," "reasoning insanity," "moral mania," or "instinctive lunacy." The challenge to psychiatry was to demonstrate that they suffered from a disease, for jurists and juries sometimes rejected medical testimony that supported a verdict of diminished responsibility. "Magistrates," the psychiatrist Henri Dagonet wrote in 1891, often "grew to doubt our science" when confronted with cases such as the following: a twenty-six-year-old man was arrested for failing to pay a bill and taken to the Sainte-Anne asylum after several years of petty crime and immoral behavior. Estranged from his respectable family, this young man seemed to be intelligent, but his conduct was highly inconsistent and suggested a "total absence of the moral sense." Besides deserting the priesthood and a wife after only fourteen days of marriage, he let a working-class woman support him and left her when her money ran out. His doctors observed that many of his crimes and indiscretions had been planned carefully; he knew what he was doing but appeared to be unable to stop himself. The contrast between his seemingly sane mind and his "inexplicable" actions baffled lay men and women, Dagonet argued, and the physician's task lay in convincing them that this was no contradiction but a symptom observed in other patients safely hospitalized in mental asylums.[40]

If two separate diagnoses of a defendant were made, medical opinions could be diametrically dissimilar because of the fluctuation of symptoms. This could lead to grave doubts about psychiatric competence, Falret told the Société on 27 March 1876. To assure that these kinds of disagreement did not arise, it was important that psychiatrists identify commonly recognized physical and psychological symptoms of reasoning insanity. Thus, alienists in the 1870s repeatedly referred to Morel's efforts to establish the physical characteristics that indicated hereditary insanity, for it was widely acknowledged that heredity was the "capital cause" of reasoning insanity and its associated mental states.[41] Falret agreed with Morel that facial asymmetry, cranial deformities, strabismus, nervous movement, paralyses, and tics were signs of a hereditary taint of the nervous system that led to mental disequilibrium and involuntarism. By including patients who exhibited these symptoms in Magnan's class of *héréditaires* and degenerates, alienists enjoyed the "principal advantage" of uniting in the same nosological category "syndromes of different symptoms," according to Magnan in 1886.[42] As another member of the Société put it, hereditary insanity was a category of mental illness into which psychiatrists could fit "everything that could not properly correspond to one of the known categories of mental pathology."[43]

Other alienists recognized these advantages. Dr. Charles Lasègue applauded Morel's class of hereditary insanity in 1873 for uniting an entire category of mental affections whose symptoms could not be associated with mania, melancholy, dementia, or idiocy. The individuals who exhibited these symptoms were the "vagabonds of insanity," Lasègue wrote, forming a pathological "caste apart." Morel's merit, he argued, lay in his examination of the ancestors of these people and his discovery in their family histories of "the numerous signs of a previous inferiority." With the identification of these symptoms as pathological, doctors could certify other individuals exhibiting the same symptoms as mentally ill.[44]

Because an alienist could cite family histories and specific physical symptoms that supposedly denoted an underlying organic cause of involuntary behavior, he stood a fair chance of proving in a court of law that the defendant was mentally ill, as Jules Falret observed in 1876.[45] The relevance of the notion of a hereditary class of the insane to forensic psychiatry was also evident to Dr. Louis Delasiauve, who noted in 1886 that for an alienist testifying that a defendant was innocent by virtue of insanity, "the verification of a hereditary predisposition" gave the psychiatrist's testimony "a decisive authority."[46] Consequently, by citing heredity and degeneracy alienists were able to extend the boundaries of mental pathology to encompass marginally deviant affective symptoms and make a plausible argument for partial insanity. Hereditarianism had the "halo" effect of convincing juries, magistrates, and the public that psychiatry was authorized to expand conventional medical taxa into areas of behavior previously managed by religion and law. [47]

If the concept of hereditary madness enjoyed a "halo of authority" that psychiatrists could exploit in courts of law, it was largely because of the growing perception in the second half of the nineteenth century that classifications of disease based on etiological principles were more scientific than those based on symptoms. In an era when alienists found it well nigh impossible to identify a single, positive cause in each case of madness, the idea that many psychological and behavioral disorders could be traced to heredity was very attractive. According to Buchez, the scientific value of Morel's method of classifying mental diseases derived from its explanation of "the genesis—not of the form—but of madness itself." It enabled the alienist to diagnose more accurately and to formulate a prognosis with a fair degree of reliability, he argued. [48] Perhaps more valuable, Morel himself added, was that a system of classifying mental illnesses that attributed many disorders to pathological heredity was similar to physicians' explanation of the etiology of other diseases and therefore reinforced the notion that alienists were bona fide physicians and that only licensed doctors should treat insanity. [49]

Equally important was the implication that the psychological disturbances intermediate between sanity and madness derived from a biophysiological deficit. According to Dr. Eugène Dally in 1869, alienists could convince magistrates and the French public of their scientific skill in identifying insanity only by aligning mental pathology more closely with pathological anatomy and physiology. [50] While Morel's list of physical symptoms indicated that reasoning insanity was characterized by certain signs, the belief that a hereditary diathesis was the primary cause of madness assured physicians of insanity's somatic pathology. As Henri Legrand du Saulle told the Société médico-psychologique on 27 March 1876, the moment alienism stopped referring to pure psychology and began examining madness from the somatic perspective, its "credit" was enhanced in the eyes of "science, justice, and the public." Those with reasoning insanity, he stressed, were *héréditaires* whose families conformed to the degenerative model Morel had described in his 1857 *Treatise*. Relying on Morel's theory of mental degeneracy, Legrand du

Saulle argued that people with a putative "lesion of the will" were recognizable by typical physical symptoms and suffered from a biological and hereditary weakness that characterized the pathological members of the human race.[51]

Hereditarianism was appropriate for mental medicine also because of the context within which nineteenth-century thinkers viewed heredity. While it was commonly acknowledged that the characteristics heredity transmitted could be both mental and physical, most thinkers agreed with Prosper Despine, a member of the Société médico-psychologique, that the reproductive process of heredity was "purely organic."[52] In 1873 Théodule Ribot declared that heredity was an essentially biophysiological process.[53] These psychologists believed that heredity explained the "automatism" or involuntary nature of deviant human behavior and thought. Ribot believed it transmitted the residues of racial experience that constituted the material basis of instinct. As both a biological force and function, heredity could account for the many instances of unconscious behavior in human beings and, according to Despine, proved that every variety of mental disturbance had a corresponding cerebral dysfunction.[54]

In his review of Ribot's book, Brierre de Boismont praised Ribot for coming to the same conclusion.[55] According to Brierre de Boismont, physiological research had demonstrated that the nervous system was "the physical condition of moral phenomena," that for every mental change there was a physical change in the substance of the brain. Normal and morbid psychological traits could be inherited just as physical attributes, such as stature and facial features, are. While both orders of characteristics were related to the biological process of heredity, neither one could be reduced to the other. For both Ribot and Brierre de Boismont, heredity was the middle term between organic matter and thought. It expressed the "ultimate identity" between the two, Brierre de Boismont wrote.[56] Heredity was another of the nineteenth-century concepts of "physiological psychology," such as reflex action, specific nerve energies, and irritability, that explained mental involuntarism in functional terms while confirming the "common sense experience of an organism as integrated body and mind."[57]

Nonetheless, the study of heredity's psychological features was by no means discredited, as Ribot's own book demonstrated. This was an important consideration for alienists who, despite rejecting the study of psychology according to its own terms,[58] were obliged as psychiatrists to refer to the patient's experienced mental state as one of the objects of medical description.[59] Mental symptoms were indispensable to the psychiatric classification of psychological diseases. The theory of degeneracy played the double role of assuring alienists of insanity's physical basis and authorizing the clinical study of the mental and behavioral signs of hereditary madness. Thus, in his 1885–1886 defense at the Société médico-psychologique of the value of hereditary insanity as a nosological category, Magnan felt comfortable discussing the clinical symptoms of degeneracy and explaining these phenomena according to recent discoveries in cerebrospinal localization.[60]

By adopting a hereditarian approach, psychiatrists could base their diagnoses on an integrated, biological relationship between body and mind without appearing less medical for recording psychopathological symptoms. Heredity was a naturalist concept of physiological psychology that excluded purely psychological interpretations of mental and nervous phenomena, but it did not reduce mind to matter. It was a felicitous "theoretical apparatus for handling the variety of communication functions in the nervous system without specifying the material or mental basis for those functions."[61] It described nervous functions of ambiguous mental or somatic status without specifying the mutual influence of mental and bodily factors. As a result, it was admissible to maintain that psychological states affected physiological operations, as Brierre de Boismont and Ribot did. This concession enabled psychiatrists to continue to attribute pathogenic significance to moral causes, a trend evident even at the height of psychiatry's so-called organicist period in the late nineteenth century.[62]

Because hereditarianism failed to specify the exact interaction between psyche and soma, it was also consistent with the form of moral treatment alienists practiced in asylums after 1850. By authorizing a vague form of psychosomatic interaction, hereditarianism allowed doctors to claim that their medical role in an asylum had an ameliorative influence on their patients. When the early nineteenth-century therapeutic optimism inspired by Philippe Pinel began to wane in midcentury, psychiatrists became less interested in the rehabilitation of the individual patient and more concerned with impersonal programs of collective psychological and behavioral modification. Alienists had less direct contact with their individual patients after midcentury and largely confined themselves to organizing the lives of asylum inmates in order to distract them from obsessional delusions.[63] This updated brand of moral treatment was managerial in nature and was more closely associated with the ethos of the regimented and overcrowded nineteenth-century asylum than either the Pinel or Leuret versions of individualized psychotherapy. It was assumed that patients would benefit from isolation in an asylum away from the often unhealthy influences of their home environments. What remained the same about post-Pinel moral treatment was the virtual identity between psychiatric moral treatment and the alienist's moral and professional integrity. Much like their British colleagues, French alienists in the nineteenth century assumed an austere pastoral responsibility for their hospitalized patients.[64] Because they exercised this responsibility almost exclusively within the asylum, their moral rectitude and probity became synonymous with the clinical, custodial, and therapeutic legitimacy of the asylum itself.

For example, in 1849 J. P. Falret argued that the asylum presented the opportunity for clinical teaching, which, despite contrary popular opinion, had a positive effect on patients and increased the doctor's authority. He argued that clinical bedside lectures in a mental hospital endowed the alienist's words with an "authority," "importance," and "solemnity" that were difficult to duplicate under other circumstances. Moreover, Falret added, the medical narration of the patient's illness before a crowd of solemn professionals was a powerful curative weapon because it objectified the disorder and convinced the patient that a new attitude was necessary—the first step, Falret claimed, toward an ultimate cure. For Falret, then, it was appropriate for the asylum alienist to impose his moral authority on his patients and to encourage the mentally disturbed to recognize the antisocial nature of their delusions.[65]

The isolation of the insane in asylums also enhanced the physician's moral authority by entrusting him with the surveillance of their conduct and thinking. As a state functionary, the asylum doctor was called upon to perform a custodial as well as therapeutic task, for the majority of his patients were viewed by the profession as potentially dangerous. The surveillance of these lunatics, Lunier maintained in 1870, was impossible outside the asylum.[66] In the asylum, Henry Bonnet wrote in 1865, the patient submitted to "moral and physical surveillance" by the physician who sought to reform the patient's ideas and instincts. The alienist assumed the role of the enlightened and virtuous penologist whose moral supervision of the insane was both benevolent and correctional.[67]

Asylum doctors appeared to be primarily concerned with managing their patients according to rigorous moral standards. The moral treatment practiced by French psychiatrists in the last century was essentially "a synthesis of medicine and morality"; when asylum doctors were not employing drugs to pacify their patients, they were advocating the "social and political norms of the time" under the guise of medical therapy.[68] Benevolence all too frequently gave way to a subtle, pernicious form of blaming the patient for being ill. Despite being raised to "the dignity of a patient,"[69] the insane were as stigmatized as ever for their inability to control their deviant behavior and thoughts through reason. Their doctors expected them to respond positively to medical appeals because, as Dr. Girard de Cailleux explained in 1861, the mad retained vestiges of their reason, no matter how debilitating their illness.[70] Doctors held a contradictory view of the lunatic as both a guiltless victim of diseased organs and the person primarily responsible for the success or failure of any moral therapy. Despite near unanimity among physicians that insanity was a somatic condition and not a result of moral failure, they still described the therapeutic effectiveness of the asylum in terms that would appease any cleric or moralist. Isolation in an asylum supposedly encouraged the patient to reflect on his or her circumstances and eventually disavow the egotism and self-indulgence that had originally led to the disorder. As was the case at Thomas Kirkbride's Pennsylvania Hospital for the Insane between 1840 and 1880, moral therapy within an asylum "took on religious overtones" because it was based on the notion that with the doctor's guidance the patient's willpower could be marshalled to control the symptoms of mental derangement. Even in the late nineteenth century, when therapeutic optimism had all but evaporated, asylum therapy implied that insanity was a moral weakness that could be cured through "repentence and willingness to reform"; it was indeed "a secularized version of the conversion experience" that in combination with the consoling aspects of moral treatment betrayed the clerical origins of many of the asylum psychiatrist's duties.[71]

Alienists' accountability for their patients' recovery was diminished by their tendency to believe that by the time a patient was entrusted to their care they could do little to reverse the physical conditions of his or her disease. This was also true for alienists' belief that the responsibility for cure was the patient's. If the patient's condition did not improve, so medical thinking went, it was because of the advanced somatic state of the illness or the lunatic's inveterate perversity—either way the alienist was blameless. Such beliefs allowed alienists to pose as "moral entrepreneurs" and recast the doctor-patient relationship in terms that benefited medicine more than the insane.[72]

Alienists particularly praised work therapy as a moralizing technique enabling the mad to acknowledge the morbid quality of their convictions and instincts. It allegedly reinforced the "communal" theme of the asylum by undermining the individualism and self-centeredness of the insane. Work, Dr. Auguste Motet said in 1864, is the "law" governing man's temporal existence. By working, Motet asserted, the insane could climb "the social ladder" and rejoin "the great human family."[73] Another psychiatrist agreed that work was the best way to diminish the patient's delirium and recreate within the asylum "the conditions of ordinary social life."[74] Dr. Bonnet explicitly explained that work therapy in mental hospitals enforced the values of society; he applauded work as a "moralizing technique" and recommended it as a way of duplicating the order of civil society and public morality within the asylum.[75]

At the center of this socialization process was the alienist and his putative moral superiority. To ensure that the insane conformed to the values of French society, the asylum doctor had to exercise complete dominion over his patients. "Without this authority and the prestige that goes with it," one alienist declared in 1884, "there is no moral treatment and, it can be added, no treatment whatsoever."[76] Lunier had been just as direct in 1870 when he told the Academy of Medicine in Paris that "it is above all in special asylums that the doctor acquires over his patients the authority without which the moral treatment is practically impossible."[77]

Despite these repeated testimonials to the palliative effects of a medically supervised moral treatment, no psychiatrist after 1860 maintained as Leuret had that the physician endeavored to cure the mind directly in moral therapy. The medical consensus was that there was no mental disease without concomitant physical injury. Therefore all therapeutic efforts had to be directed initially toward curing the diseased brain of the patient. Yet psychiatrists also believed that the insane benefited immeasurably from exposure through hospitalization to the psychological process of normalization. They were convinced that incarceration in a medical institution free of the intellectual and emotional stress of the patient's domestic and occupational environment encouraged self-control and peace of mind. At the same time, alienists agreed that moral treatment could only achieve this goal by first restoring the lunatic's thinking organ to health. By undermining the insane's hallucinations and illusions, the doctor paved the way toward the stabilization of the material conditions of the brain.[78] As Bonnet wrote in 1865, isolation in an asylum achieved cures of insanity by engendering "calm in the organism."[79]

How did psychiatrists reconcile psychological treatment with somatic disease? One way was to ignore the paradox, another was to minimize the dualistic distinction between mind and body, making it possible to imagine a close, causal connection between the two. In 1855 Emile Renaudin admitted that one could refer to a body and mind in psychological medicine but maintained that they were inseparable in pathology and that there was a clear "psychosomatic" relationship between them.[80] If it were thought that body and mind were integrally related at a fundamental level, then the notion that moral treatment had a beneficial influence on the nervous system would be acceptable.[81]

Hereditarianism in the form of degeneracy theory accounted for the alleged efficacy of asylum-based moral treatment. Morel declared that it was virtually impossible to disentangle the complex interaction of body and mind. Even when a physical cause was identified in a specific case of insanity, he wrote in 1846, its influence on the mental faculties could not be sufficiently isolated to permit one to say that it was the "exclusive organic cause acting independently of every intellectual and moral element."[82] He later explained that although biological heredity was responsible for the pathological organic predisposition of the nervous system in degeneracy, the resulting neurological lesion was diffuse and unlocalized in most cases and could be attributed to a variety of psychological and physical causes, none of which in itself could have produced mental derangement. As an example he cited the immoral life-style frequently observed among alcoholics' parents, circumstances which he believed were as etiologically important as the pathophysiological conditions of alcoholic intoxication. In his treatise on degeneracy Morel proposed the "law of double fecundation," which attributed equal significance to moral elements and to organic conditions in the development of mental degeneracy.[83] Medical moral treatment was vital to help to counteract the inherited organic conditions of madness. If psychological and physical forces combined to produce a functional neuropathic lesion that became a hereditary organic disposition to madness in the next generation, then psychological conditioning through asylum isolation was a legitimate means of reducing somatic deficit. Hereditarianism in the degenerative context enabled psychiatrists to "smooth . . . away the logical awkwardness of employing 'moral' means to treat a physical disease" while retaining the dualist notions of psyche and soma.[84] Hereditarianism was a scientific rationale based on the moral and pedagogical authority of asylum alienists for the use of collective psychotherapy to modify the cerebrovascular state of the insane.

Morel's theory of hereditary degeneracy was useful because it not only explained how therapy in the milieu of the asylum redeemed the moral authority of the alienist but also cast the alienist as the expert in social matters and public mental health. Morel proposed that the environment and routine of the mental hospital serve as the model for reorganizing social life and restoring the French nation to health. Like many of his colleagues in mental medicine, he was shaken in the 1860s by the public suspicion of the asylum's usefulness. He acknowledged that asylums had filled up with "an enormous mass of incurables," patients suffering from chronic mental illness, paralytic insanity, and senile dementia.[85] He agreed that these conditions made it almost impossible for doctors to fulfill their therapeutic responsibilities but denied that the therapeutic ethos of the asylum was necessarily at fault. On the contrary, he and other alienists blamed the public and lay administrators for institutionalizing the insane only when their diseases became chronic, a practice that psychiatrists alleged led to overcrowding. What was necessary, Morel wrote in 1857, was the extension of the asylum's techniques of hygiene, behavior modification, and moral instruction to society itself to eliminate the social factors that caused insanity. No longer, he wrote, were alienists concerned only with the psychological welfare of single patients but also with public health.[86] Just as alienists taught their hospitalized patients to accept civic responsibilities and the "duties dictated by the fixed and immutable moral and divine law," so the French "masses" ought to be educated according to these same medical guidelines for mental health. Morel advocated a "moralization of the masses" because he feared that the "fallen classes" of the industrial proletariat and rural poor would descend the anthropological ladder even farther unless the degenerative conditions of their lives were substantially improved.[87]

When Morel referred to a crisis of the asylum at midcentury, his fellow alienists understood, for they were also disturbed by growing public complaints that asylums were sites of medical futility and unwarranted incarceration. If they agreed with Morel's new system for classifying mental diseases or if they identified clinical syndromes such as moral insanity and reasoning insanity as the effects of morbid heredity, it was largely because these classes of mental alienation implied that the public's failure to recognize madness unaccompanied by manic delirium or total loss of reason was responsible for the problems psychiatrists had curing their patients. This failure had two likely consequences, according to hereditarian thinking: it postponed the hospitalization of insane persons until it was too late to cure them; and it gave them more opportunity to reproduce, thereby multiplying the numbers of degenerates, increasing the eventual costs of public assistance to the insane, and making the task of psychiatry all the harder. Only by combining a stricter institutionalization policy with a campaign for moral reform among the pauper and working classes, many alienists argued, could the crisis in asylum treatment be solved. "That is your task," one psychiatrist advised his lay readers in 1866, "and that is your remedy." The asylum itself remained blameless.[88]

Morel's program for the moral regeneration of French society had a politically manipulative tone, as Brierre de Boismont pointed out.[89] Morel hoped to correct "the absence of an attitude of duty," "the perversion of religious sentiment," and the seeming unwillingness of the lower classes to distinguish good from evil—conditions, he claimed, that characterized "the dangerous classes" that threatened all civilized nations.[90] However, Morel's aim in endorsing this program of moral regeneration was professional as well as political. As he stated in his treatise on degeneracy, one of his principal goals was to prove that medicine's moral therapy could be applied on a far greater scale than previously imagined.[91] In recommending that psychiatrically approved psychological treatment be used to solve the moral problems of society, Morel sought to establish that alienists could serve as health consultants to governmental policy makers and as the sole authorities in "the positive indication of remedies" for curing the virtual epidemic of mental disease. By achieving this recognition of their expertise in public mental health, Morel added, alienists could refute their detractors who accused psychiatry of therapeutic "impotence."[92]

Morel intended his hereditarian theory of degeneracy to shift public criticism from psychiatry's dubious record of cure and questionable therapeutic methods to the morally unwholesome social, economic, and cultural environment. He hoped that his ideas would ensure medicine's credentials as a guardian of morality within the asylum and as an authority on public morality outside the asylum. Morel foresaw alienists attacking the sentiments he identified as responsible for the spiritual bankruptcy of the lower classes. Morel explicitly advocated the use of the term *moral treatment* to designate the method of education necessary to coax the poor away from their vices, such as their supposed fondness for alcohol.[93] And because the phrase *moral treatment* was "deeply rooted in the classical asylum tradition,"[94] the image of the public mental hospital as a utilitarian social institution could be improved and its shortcomings disguised. Morel had deftly turned the widespread reappraisal of the asylum into a reaffirmation of its basic characteristics and imperatives.

Moral education by asylum doctors was only part of a wider program of "moral and physical hygiene." In addition to primary education, the sexual mores of the working class, and the crime and suicide rates, Morel felt psychiatrists also ought to be concerned with the great variety of toxic agents in the air and in food in French industrial areas, which combined with moral depravity to produce degeneracy. Morel identified tobacco, hashish, lead, and ergot as poisonous elements in the environment,[95] but directed most of his attention to another physical cause of degeneracy: alcoholic intoxication. It and the inadequate diet of the lower classes were the two most important physical causes of degeneracy, according to Morel.[96] He, like many of his colleagues, believed that the offspring of alcoholics could inherit a predisposition to drunkenness or acquire a taste for liquor from its mother during the fetal and nursing stages. Once acquired, alcoholism set in motion the hereditary sequence leading to the eventual sterility of certain families.

Morel was convinced that as a "moral entrepreneur" the alienist should become an authority on the mental health of families. If the scourge of nineteenth-century French society was morbid heredity, then medical supervision of family planning was imperative. As he pointed out in 1857, breeding experiments with plants and animals as well as the history of civilization indicated that the most serious threat to the health and longevity of racial groups was consanguinity, or intermarriage within the same gene pool.[97] The consequences were evident in pathology, Morel argued, for he claimed that his studies of degeneracy had revealed that abnormal mental states could often be traced to marriages between spouses with unhealthy family histories. Morel believed that the alienist should focus on "the hygiene of the family," regulating the psychosocial and physical conditions of families and advising them on medically proper marriage partners.[98]

Morel's refrain of psychiatric expertise in family hygiene struck a responsive chord within mental medicine. For example, his student Doutrebente wrote in 1868 that hereditarian studies had shown that hygienically unwise marriages led to the degeneration of the families and thus to the degeneration of the human race itself. In his conclusion, endorsed by Morel,[99] Doutrebente stressed the alienist's duty to "penetrate to the bosom of families and endeavor to conquer the scruples and the secrets of pusillanimous people who under a more or less valid pretext, seek to divert the doctor from the truth and often lead him completely to error." Appealing to the duty of science to render service to society by approving suitable marriages on the basis of sound heredity, Doutrebente chastised the French public for refusing to divulge information on the health of family members. The resistance to medical interrogation of family members was, in his opinion, contrary to their own interests and the interests of society.[100]

In 1869 Auguste Motet endorsed Doutrebente's conclusions and cited Ulysée Trélat's 1861 book on lucid insanity as further support for the notion that if human reproduction were not medically monitored, the nation and the human race might be doomed. Referring to Morel's ideas, Motet observed that while degenerative families eventually died out because of sterility, their biological descent all too often dragged the "sane of mind" down with them.[101] Hence, according to the emerging psychiatric view, families tainted with hereditary degeneracy constituted a threat to society as well as to themselves, and their plight warranted medical management.

Trélat believed that the future of marriage as a social institution was in peril because hereditary considerations were ignored. He implored people to base their decisions to marry on "the constitution, health, intelligence, and the moral qualities of the family with which you propose to contract an alliance" and not on the wealth such a marriage would bring. To ignore medical advice in this matter only served to debase marriage, "the highest and holiest institution of all human institutions."[102] In view of such sentiments, it is little wonder that other doctors foresaw a noble future for mental medicine recording family histories in order to prevent hygienically inappropriate marriages. For example, Dr. Durand de Gros told the Société médico-psychologique that by studying "the natural history of the hereditary diatheses," doctors would learn what moral and physical elements caused "the pathological plague [of degeneracy] that, while it devoured en masse present-day generations, at the same time assured itself of rich prey in those of the future." At the root of this process, he declared, were marriages between relatives or people with histories of disease, a social phenomenon he felt alienists were especially qualified to regulate. Echoing Morel's call to concentrate on social groups such as the family rather than isolated individuals, Durand de Gros encouraged alienists to eliminate the "parasitic germs" that flowed in the blood of some families, the most constructive step toward stemming the debilitating hereditary neuropathic epidemic that threatened future generations.[103]

Alienists may well have been sincere in their intentions to improve family mental health, but they were also aware of the professional advantages of a policy of family hygiene. Striking at the root of hereditary degeneracy through family medicine was one way to reduce the numbers of chronically ill patients in French asylums and therefore to combat the public image of mental hospitals as "factories of incurability." As one Bicêtre physician wrote in 1866, psychiatrists ought to supervise all aspects of family life relating to health: diet, housing, morality, physical fitness, alcoholic consumption, domestic and occupational stress, and the choice of spouse.[104] Similarly, Henri Girard de Cailleux recommended that alienists follow Morel's plan of eliminating the physical and psychological causes of degeneracy through an active policy of "social hygiene" aimed at the family.[105]

Growing psychiatric interest in family mental health was an indication of the alienist alignment with the burgeoning hygiene movement within French medicine. Alienists had been associated with the hygiene movement since the founding of the *Annales d'hygiène publique et de médecine légale* in 1829.[106] For the most part they had felt that their asylum activities were consistent with the goals of public mental health, but the appearance of Morel's book on degeneracy in 1857 signaled a change in psychiatric attitudes. Asylum doctors increasingly expressed their disenchantment with the therapeutic alternatives of hospital medicine and their willingness to serve more effectively as state functionaries in areas such as family hygiene. The tendency of psychiatrists to embrace this task was overdetermined by the material and social conditions of medical practice in the nineteenth century. For example, when physicians realized that the severe overcrowding of the profession in the 1830s and 1840s had produced significant unemployment, they cast their eyes on the opportunities for employment as medical representatives of government in the field of public health.[107] Family hygiene looked promising for alienists because of the social interest in the welfare of the family, interest that intensified after 1848.[108] The application of hygienic principles to family life-style was seen as a way of improving the reproductive conditions and the health of the race.[109] At the same time, hygienic medicine enabled alienists to rationalize their loss of confidence in conventional "heroic therapy" while authorizing their new roles as "medical police." Hygienists had already pointed out the advantages of public medicine for physicians: prophylactic measures offered more therapeutic alternatives than "the pharmaceutical arsenal," one doctor wrote in 1844.[110] Physicians felt that preventive steps through the strict regulation of public health were professionally preferable to traditional curative procedures.[111]

This feature of hygiene had a patent appeal to psychiatry, whose therapeutic record was a source of considerable public embarrassment. As Morel admitted in 1857, of all physicians alienists particularly felt the need to shift the study of treatment "onto a terrain more fertile with results." The therapeutic resources of hospital psychiatry were far too limited to stem the social tide of insanity, he argued.[112] Similarly, Durand de Gros lamented in 1868 that medicine's role had been principally restricted to "the barbarous practice" of treating "one by one the bad weeds that infest the field of human health." However, he said, by practicing the benevolent and socially utilitarian methods of prophylactic medicine on the family and not "therapeutics properly speaking," the future would be rosy for alienism.[113]

Through their espousal of degeneracy theory and hereditarianism alienists were able to depict themselves as experts in family hygiene and to sidestep the question of their competence and the asylum's obsolescence as a therapeutic institution. Degeneracy theory diverted attention from the medical skill of alienism to the myriad physical and psychological forces in society that caused hereditary insanity, thereby undercutting the arguments of those who viewed psychiatrists as responsible for the high incidence of madness. The irony is that alienists tried to gain credence as medical specialists and public health experts by reaffirming the ideals of the asylum, the locus of their futile therapies for over half a century and the target of antipsychiatric sentiment. They addressed a serious challenge to their identity as medical practitioners by maintaining that the source of psychiatry's woes was really the solution. Having been accused of exercising unwarranted power in public asylums, institutional psychiatrists contended that they needed even more authority in order to eradicate the roots of mental disease, despite a history that belied their ability to do so.

Nevertheless, alienist reliance on degeneracy theory was largely rhetorical. While Morel recommended psychiatric participation in social programs designed to eradicate the causes of mental degeneracy, the bulk of alienists preferred to concentrate on the administration of madness in public asylums. The one notable exception was the temperance movement, the beginnings of which Morel had applauded in 1857.[114] When the Société française de tempérance was founded in 1872, over one-third of its members were physicians. The alienist Ludger Lunier was a leading figure in this organization. But although it helped to create the medical and political interest in the dangers of drunkenness that led to the "Roussel law" of 3 February 1873—which made it a crime to be intoxicated in public[115]—the Société française de tempérance "plainly lacked vitality and seems to have had no substantial popular following." A vigorous temperance movement thrived in England in the last century, but "French soil proved extremely inhospitable to any such organization."[116] At the turn of the century Clemenceau observed that French temperance had few positive accomplishments.

Even with regard to the obvious eugenic implications of hereditarianism, most alienists were reluctant to encourage legislative steps to avert the consequences of intermarriage between lunatics. Despite the alienist belief that neuropaths were sexually attracted to each other,[117] Charles Féré could still maintain as late as 1895 that "a law prohibiting the marriage of certain categories of degenerates" was impractical because degenerates would not submit to such a law.[118] More important, to diagnose someone as an unmitigated hereditary danger to the human race was to admit that the individual was incurably insane, which was to admit the powerlessness of psychiatry, something alienists did not like to do. This consideration surfaced during the debates over the Ferry government's divorce bill between 1881 and 1884. While some alienists, like Eugène Dally and Jean Luys, endorsed the proposed clause in the bill that named insanity as a reason for divorce, the majority within the medical community disagreed. Physicians like Charcot, Magnan, and Legrand du Saulle believed that although hereditary predisposition was a highly important factor in the production of insanity, it did not always signify incurability. In part because of this opinion, the original insanity clause was dropped from the divorce bill.[119] When on 29 January 1883 the Société médico-psychologique discussed whether someone with mentally ill parents was fatally insane, Dr. Eugène Billod emphasized that if a hereditarily predisposed individual consistently and carefully followed hygienic principles and avoided stresses, then there was no necessary incurability.[120] Because alienists wanted to be recognized as experts whose advice on questions of family and public mental health was authoritative, they disliked categorical definitions of mental illness that made the opinions of physicians appear superfluous. In hereditarianism they discovered the model of mental illness that under the guise of science mystified the diagnosis and treatment of madness and reinforced the sense of "legitimate complexity" surrounding the practice of psychological medicine.[121] This psychiatric attitude was the same in 1887 as it had been in 1867; alienists felt that they and not inflexible laws should decide matters relating to the hereditary predisposition to madness.[122]

It would be a mistake to view pre-1900 alienists as deeply interested in what is today called "social psychiatry." In using the terminology of degeneracy theory, they seemed more preoccupied with legitimizing existing psychiatric practices than with carving out new social territories for medical intervention. Although alienists sounded like early twentieth-century psychiatrists who looked beyond the asylum for opportunities to practice their craft, they differed from their successors because they were primarily interested in defending rather than reforming hospital services for the insane. With the exception of legal medicine, the psychiatric horizon was limited to the asylum. Degeneracy theory did for French psychiatry at a particularly difficult time in its history what phrenology did for English psychiatry between 1820 and 1840: it "legitimat[ed] the humanitarianism and utilitarianism" of hospital moral treatment "while simultaneously justifying" the presence of alienists in asylums "as the purveyors of essential medical expertise."[123] Degeneracy theory conformed to the observation that medical theories are often "rationalizations to justify the use of methods and materials that are much older than the theory."[124] Quite simply, hereditarianism's value to psychiatry lay less in its capacity to improve medical asylum practice than in its potential for sustaining the image of alienists as experts in the institutional management of madness.

Chapter Seven

Science, Politics, and Psychiatric Hereditarianism in the Nineteenth Century

With the advent of hereditarianism in the 1860s, alienists began the intellectual struggle to vindicate themselves as medically useful asylum physicians. Yet alienists longed to be recognized not just as institutional "moral entrepreneurs" but also as positivist *scientists*. The rhetorical form of hereditarianism and degeneracy theory was appropriate for their purposes because it blended biomedically and culturally congruent themes into a hegemonic body of knowledge that reassured Republican officials of their dedication to the positivist goals of progress and order. Psychiatric hereditarianism and degeneracy theory imposed an ideologically acceptable logic on madness and other pressing social problems. By adopting hereditarianism alienists could depict the psychiatrist as a scientist endowed with moral authority and committed to naturalism, secularism, the defense of the family and private property, and the progress of civilization.[1] Alienism could also hope to improve its relations with the state and undermine "the notion of alienists as *alienated*," that is, to erase the image of the psychiatrist as someone who, like the people he treated, lived inside the walls of the asylum and beyond the pale of everyday society.[2]

Hereditarianism in the form of degeneracy theory was especially suitable for alienists who sought to strengthen psychiatry's ties to mainstream medicine, which had already shown considerable interest in the question of heredity. As early as 1840 the internist Dr. P.

A. Piorry remarked on the tendency of doctors as well as authors of medical theses at the Paris Faculty of Medicine to view heredity as the principal predisposition to chronic and constitutional diseases.[3] For the alienist Achille Foville in 1860, heredity was "the great fact . . . that dominates in all its grandeur so many important medical questions."[4] Three years later Jean Luys observed in his medical thesis that since Piorry's book in 1840 there had been many theses about the influence of heredity on scrofula, tuberculosis, cancer, syphilis, gout, and nervous disorders.[5] Similarly, in an 1864 article in the *Annales médico-psychologiques*, the English doctor Hugh Grainger-Steward remarked that "the hereditary transmission of diseases, or a tendency to contract them, has attracted much more attention in the last few years than previously."[6]

There was lively medical interest at midcentury in the effects of heredity on the incidence of nervous disease. As Dr. Edmond Dupouy noted in 1865, heredity was considered to be a special characteristic of nervous affections.[7] In 1845 the Academy of Medicine in Paris had awarded a prize to the best essay on this topic.[8] Many of the contestants argued that because neurological disturbances often existed independently of organic structural injury to the nervous system, these disturbances were probably caused by changing levels of nervous energy or *névrosité*. When certain stimuli impinged on the nervous system, specific reactions would occur according to the pre-established functional relation between nervous tissue and the arterial blood. Any lack of harmony in this relationship was attributed to a hereditary cause.[9]

Jacques Moreau de Tours was one alienist who favored the notion of heredity as the cause of nervous disturbances.[10] Insanity was already considered to be a chronic disease of the nervous system; by attributing it to a hereditary diffuse neuropathic diathesis, alienists could cite a conventional pathological concept, explain away the absence of any signs of localized organic lesions, and associate mental alienation with other documented, functional diseases of the nervous system.

Hereditarian ideas became even more appealing to alienists with the rise of the "Charcot school" of neuropathology at the Salpêtrière after 1870.[11] By 1882, when Gambetta appointed him to the first chair in the diseases of the nervous system at the Faculty of Medicine, Jean Martin Charcot was at the height of his fame. He had made a string of impressive discoveries in pathological neuroanatomy since becoming a ward head at Salpêtrière in 1862. After 1870 he turned to the study of hysteria, and in the late 1870s, hypnosis. Charcot believed that a neuropathic hereditary taint was extremely important in hysteria.[12] Jules Dejerine, a member of the Charcot school, wrote a treatise in 1886 in which he conjectured that all illnesses of the nervous system had a common origin in the hereditary transmission of a flawed nervous condition that could manifest itself in many different ways. According to Dejerine, these illnesses were divided into two basic pathological groups. One group included the nervous disorders without anatomical lesions, such as hysteria, neurasthenia, and epilepsy. The other group included the nervous disorders with anatomical lesions, such as general paralysis and locomotor ataxia.[13] Charles Féré, another pupil of Charcot, also expanded his teacher's ideas with his theory of "the neuropathic family," a single category that combined mental and neurological diseases on the basis of hereditary predisposition. Féré, too, linked insanity to somatic neurological diseases like tuberculosis and general paresis, adding them to this family of neuropathic illnesses.[14]

It was in the interests of psychiatry to emphasize neuropathic heredity in mental illness. By stressing hereditarianism, alienists could call attention to the links between insanity and neurological diseases with identifiable organic lesions, thereby reinforcing the physicalist nature of mental alienation, which psychiatrists considered to be crucial to the defence of their therapeutic prerogatives. For example, a series of articles in the *Annales médico-psychologiques* in February 1887 cited the work of Charcot, Féré, and Dejerine as confirming that the incidence of mental alienation, hysteria, neuropathy, cancer, arthritis, rickets, and other constitutional diseases was extremely high in families tainted by bad heredity.[15] The Charcot school's emphasis on nervous heredity had been brought to the attention of the Société officially on 10 December 1883 by Dr. Landouzy and Dr. Ballet, both followers of Charcot. They described how Charcot attributed locomotor ataxia—the tertiary stage of syphilis—to a "hereditary nervous predisposition" and not to an infectious source. Because of its hereditary origin, Landouzy and Ballet announced, ataxia belonged to the "great family of affections of the nervous system" and constituted a topic that was "right at home in the Société médico-psychologique."[16]

Increased alienist interest in nervous heredity during the 1880s was in part attributable to the influence of Charcot and his pupils in neurology. Since the early nineteenth century many alienists— Lasègue and Moreau to name two—had studied the less debilitating forms of nervous illnesses, like hysteria, and most asylum psychiatrists had seen their share of hysterical patients.[17] However, in 1878 and 1882 the republican state divided this medical field, customarily psychiatry's purview, into two different chairs at the Faculty of Medicine, one for the mental diseases and one for the diseases of the nervous system. The division was disquieting for psychiatrists because it implied a status difference between a discipline that dealt with elusive mental maladies and an emerging medical specialty that succeeded far more than psychiatry in correlating clinical symptoms with organic lesions. Close relations between Charcot's followers and alienists like Féré represented for the latter a narrowing of the troublesome gap that threatened to widen at any time. Yet, equally important was the republican regime's tacit endorsement of Charcot's work by creating for him the chair in nervous diseases. For a profession still smarting from its association with the discredited Bonapartists, alienism would have been eager to curry favor with Gambetta and the republicans by publicizing the similarities between psychiatric thinking and the theories of the Charcot school.

There were other features of psychiatric hereditarianism whose consistency with developments in biomedical science alienists were eager to point out. For example, Morel in his 1857 treatise on degeneracy had praised Claude Bernard's studies of the effects of toxic substances on the organism's functions as a vital contribution to an understanding of how poisonous elements in the environment disrupted physiological operations; this disruption was the first step, Morel believed, in the pathological sequence leading to degeneracy.[18] In pointing out these similarities, Morel was also making the larger point that the alienist interpretation of a neuropathic lesion as functional and nonlocalized was consistent with the physiological definition of a lesion as anatomically independent of a specific organ.[19]

Still other developments in French biomedical science served to popularize hereditarianism in psychiatry. Between 1843 and 1870 the physiologist C. E. Brown-Séquard performed numerous experiments to study the hereditary transmission of the effects of certain injuries to the nervous system of guinea pigs. He discovered that by deliberately injuring the nervous system he could produce epilepsy. He also claimed that the progeny of these epileptic guinea pigs became epileptic themselves and concluded that each offspring inherited "the morbid state" of its mother's or father's nervous system, the predisposition of the nervous system to disease.[20]

Alienists were quick to grasp the importance of Brown-Séquard's experiments. In January 1868 Achille Foville read a paper to the Société médico-psychologique on the hereditary transmission of epilepsy and cited Brown-Séquard's work on guinea pigs.[21] In his 1873 book on hereditary insanity, Henri Legrand du Saulle also cited Brown-Séquard's experiments, as did Charles Féré in 1884.[22] Brown-Séquard's experiments were interesting to alienists because they suggested that acquired pathological characteristics could be inherited, an important consideration given that Lamarckianism prevailed in French biology during the second half of the century. Darwin's theory of natural selection made little headway in French science because of the fierce chauvinist allegiance to the transformist ideas of the eighteenth-century naturalist Jean Baptiste Lamarck. French neo-Lamarckianism viewed evolution as mediated between the internal physiology of an organism and its environment. Successful adaptation depended on the ability of the organism to adjust to changing environmental conditions. The characteristics that led to successful adaptation were then passed on to the next generation. However, successful adaptation to a particular environment in the short run periodically proved to be harmful to the organism in the long run, the pathological consequences only becoming evident in later generations.[23] Degeneracy theory was the medical counterpart to Lamarckian biology. It explained how physical and mental disorders could result over several generations from accommodation to a pathogenic environment, such as the industrial region around Rouen, where Morel practiced as an alienist. By studying mental pathology from the standpoint of degeneracy and morbid heredity, alienists could demonstrate their allegiance to the reigning principle of French biology.

Biological considerations punctuated much of psychiatric writing after midcentury. One example was the 1868 article on reasoning insanity by Dr. Campagne of the Montdevergues asylum (Vaucluse). Despite widespread rejection of Darwinism and spon-

taneous generation as a materialist theory, Campagne argued that
natural selection was the decisive factor in the etiology of partial
insanity. Acting with heredity, Campagne maintained, natural selection eliminated those with bad health as unfit for the struggle for
existence. Yet, aware of the potentially unorthodox implications of
his ideas, Campagne muted the Darwinist element in his reasoning.[24] He stressed that "the law of selection" could be accepted
independently of Darwin's theory. There was nothing in Campagne's espousal of natural selection that was necessarily inconsistent with the Lamarckian orientation of degeneracy theory, for both
Morel and Magnan considered the products of mental degeneracy
to be hereditarily unnatural and a danger to the human race.

Campagne also took the opportunity to point out that the
achievements of experimental medicine had demonstrated that organic responses to certain environmental stimuli followed identifiable laws. "This great principle of proportionality between causes
and effects" in physiology linked biology to the mechanistic physical
sciences, he continued, and could be applied to the study of mental
pathology.[25] Campagne apparently believed that this principle of
proportionality constituted a common ground on which psychiatry,
biology, and the physical sciences could be allied. His article revealed how psychiatrists sought to erase the gap between alienism
and the so-called hard sciences. Biological ideas based on the impla-
cable force of inheritance were ideal for this purpose, for as the
experimental psychologist Théodule Ribot wrote in 1873, "heredity
is but one form of that ultimate law which by physicists is called the
conservation of energy and by metaphysicians universal causality."[26] Hereditarianism was a felicitous way for alienists to appear
scientifically up-to-date in the second half of the nineteenth century.

While alienists did not hesitate to use hereditarianism to associate psychiatry with the most recent themes of biomedical science,
they realized that their hereditarian approach to mental illness
maintained a link with the past. Late nineteenth-century hereditarianism may have contained many novel features, but it was not
new. When writing on heredity, physicians rarely failed to men-
tion that heredity's role in the development of disease had been
recognized throughout the history of medicine. In 1860 Albert
Mitivié, son of the prominent alienist Jules Mitivié (1796–1871),

wrote that the modern notion of hereditary predisposition to illness could be traced to such venerable thinkers of antiquity as
Pythagoras and Hippocrates.[27]

In 1864 Hugh Grainger-Steward also cited Hippocrates as well as
Fernal, Burton, Paracelsus, and Bruno as early writers on heredity.
For Grainger-Steward and his French colleagues, the idea of morbid heredity had grown naturally out of medical concepts such as
"temperament" and "constitution" that were tied to the humoral
tradition. For example, it had long been held that psychological
characteristics were related to underlying physical constitution.
Since antiquity physicians had frequently examined both the patient's medical history and that of his or her ancestors in order to
clarify diagnosis and prognosis. Precursors of nineteenth-century
hereditarianism, Grainger-Steward pointed out, had even anticipated essentially modern notions such as the proscription of marriages among insane, gouty, or epileptic persons.[28]

Their acceptance of hereditarianism, then, made psychiatrists
appear to be at once traditional, progressive, and guided by common sense. So compelling was the evidence that some healthy or
unhealthy mental and physical characteristics were inherited that
Jules Baillarger conceded that even before the "fact" of hereditary
predisposition had been embraced by science "it had already become popular."[29]

Public awareness of a hereditary component to mental illness was
evidenced further at the 30 December 1867 meeting of the Société
médico-psychologique, at which Baillarger said that twice in the
past year he had been consulted by people concerned that their
children would develop a neuropathic disease because other family
members had nervous or psychological problems.[30] How much
public concern with morbid heredity stemmed from medical efforts
to publicize the topic is difficult to say. However, Baillarger's admission that physicians' knowledge of the topic was hardly more
refined than the public's suggests that they had only recently paid
attention to it. Baillarger's advice that medicine gather more information on morbid heredity in order to answer the public's questions
also suggests that some alienists viewed hereditarianism as having
so much popular currency that mental medicine had to address it in
order to appear authoritative. Such was the case when the issue
arose again on 29 January 1883 when Dr. Eugène Billod read a

paper to the Société on the appropriate alienist response to the question of whether a person with insane parents was likely to fall mentally ill. The ensuing debate focused on the curability of patients with bad heredity, but the more fundamental issue was medical expertise. What was an alienist to say when asked if bad heredity was fatal? As Billod recounted, he was sometimes confronted with the popular belief that madness was a disease of the blood and therefore hereditary; he advised hereditarily predisposed individuals to strictly follow the guidelines of moral and physical hygiene. The content of such advice is less important than alienists' belief that they had to respond to questions about morbid heredity if they wished to maintain a semblance of professional expertise.[31]

Alienists' attention to hereditary matters was also related to French society's larger preoccupation with the possible pathological consequences of reproduction. Since the 1840s an increasing number of political, literary, and scientific figures had expressed concern about the future of France as a distinctive racial and national community. Whether the prognosis was optimistic or pessimistic, virtually all major thinkers agreed that France at midcentury was at a crossroads politically, socially, morally, and biologically. When the alienist profession fully embraced hereditarianism in the 1880s, a passionate debate in medicine and lay society had been raging for at least thirty years over the biological fitness and political future of the Gallic race.

The public hygiene movement in French medicine in the first half of the nineteenth century had produced an avalanche of statistics that documented the poor physical and mental health of the working class of France's burgeoning industrial centers. Even before Morel popularized the term *degeneracy*, writers were commenting on the "degeneration" of the population in the large cities of France.[32] The shocking evidence of disease and socioeconomic injustice led physicians to believe that the future of medicine lay in identifying the living conditions that would stem the apparent decline in urban health and fitness. After midcentury medical attention became fixated on the formidable task of reversing this deterioration. Poor reproductive practices were quickly identified as a major cause of ill health, and a vast medical literature emerged on the dangers of marrying someone with a poor family medical history. Beginning in the 1850s and throughout the next decade physicians also debated the health risks of marrying a relative. This debate was fueled by the writings on family hygiene of physicians such as Eugène Bouchut, Francis Devay, J. B. Dehoux, Prosper Menière, and Jean Boudin, which received a great deal of attention in the *Annales d'hygiène publique et de médecine légale*, the organ of the French hygienist movement in medicine.[33] The debate over the medically proper conditions of reproduction frequently encompassed not only the health of French families but also the health of entire population groups, such as the population of Paris.[34]

By 1867 the topic of France's degeneration and decline in fitness was au courant enough to prompt the Academy of Medicine to discuss the problem at a series of meetings from March to July 1867. Most participants accepted that the French populace was significantly older and less fertile than those of other countries, although few agreed that national decline was inevitable. The consensus was that there was "danger for the future" if sufficient attention were not paid to the "productive and intrinsic worth" of the French people, as one physician put it. This collective concern with the relative quality of the population explained why so many physicians in the 1850s and 1860s were interested in the reproductive practices and hereditary histories of French families.[35]

If many physicians had become increasingly convinced that the study of reproduction and heredity explained the declining vitality and fertility of the nation, many nonmedical savants, intellectuals, and literary figures tended to share their opinion that France's future was gloomy unless drastic measures were taken.[36] Political events after 1848 sharpened this fear. The collapse of the "experiment" of the Second Republic (1848–1851) led liberals such as Philippe Buchez and Ernest Renan to think that progress, seemingly inexorable in the 1840s, was highly questionable. Spokespersons for the political right tended to concur, citing the 1848 Revolution and its course of events as proof that democratic reforms— like the expansion of the franchise during the Second Empire from 240,000 to nine million voters—were bound to end in chaos and conflict or, as one observer wrote in 1860, "turbulent decadence."[37]

The preoccupation with national decadence intensified after the Franco-Prussian War and the Paris Commune of 1871. The Commune was an independent revolutionary government established in Paris from 18 March to 28 May 1871. The new republican government crushed the Commune in a single week during which twenty to twenty-five thousand people were killed or executed. Since most of the Parisians who resisted were from the lower classes, one of the more immediate effects of the Commune was that bourgeois attitudes toward the pauper classes hardened. "From the anguish of foreign and civil war emerged the myth, sturdy and none too subtle, of the habitually drunken, politically dangerous commoner."[38] This new myth of the proletarian as a politically irresponsible dipsomaniac reinforced conventional ideas of the degenerate and dangerous nature of the lower classes, their congenital immaturity for democracy, and their contribution to the increasing civil instability of France since the 1789 Revolution.[39]

Other ideological reactions to the *année terrible* of 1870–1871 strengthened the belief that France was a decadent nation. France's defeat at the hands of Germany suggested to many French thinkers that Germany's rise could only be sustained in Europe by the corresponding decline of its neighbor across the Rhine. The presence of Germany after 1870 was the very symbol of France's fall from diplomatic, intellectual, moral, and demographic power. Unified Germany in 1870 had a larger population than France, a higher birthrate, and a greater capacity for economic growth and even seemed to be outstripping France in theoretical and applied science.[40]

Bourgeois optimism was also chilled by the significant decline of industrial activity and investment after 1882. French agriculture, staggered by the phylloxera epidemic that peaked in the 1880s, suffered in the second half of the nineteenth century. As a result, workers migrated to the cities from the countryside in search of jobs that became increasingly scarce as economic stagnation set in.[41] Dislocation and urban unemployment fostered political discontent that ultimately led to the election of fifty socialist deputies in 1893, an event that shook what little bourgeois complacency might have remained in fin de siècle France. These symptoms of economic crisis[42] combined with the political scandals and turbulence of the 1880s and 1890s to encourage a discourse of decline, decadence, and degeneracy that continued until the nationalist revival of 1905–1914.[43] A literature of decadence, a movement that began in the years 1880–1885, flourished in the last two decades of the century.[44] Although literary fascination with decadence was not unprecedented in France,[45] the explosion of interest in it at the end of the century indicated that French writers were self-consciously exploring the forms of expression appropriate for a civilization they deemed to be in its dying stages.[46] Literary disillusionment with the world articulated the general crisis of faith in France's future.

The hereditarian rhetoric of psychiatrists throughout the last third of the nineteenth century not only reflected these cultural concerns and anxieties but also refracted them in a way that served the interests of mental medicine by making alienists appear to be experts on the problems of social solidarity and national unity. Since the beginning of the century psychiatrists had been eager to play the role of political commentators.[47] After midcentury, hereditarianism and degeneration punctuated much of their political commentary. The first alienist to contend that heredity had an important bearing on a wide range of political and social issues was Prosper Lucas, who commented in 1847 on the unprecedented interest in the question of heredity and attributed it to the challenge that the Saint-Simonian, Fourierist, and communist movements presented to the legitimacy of the family, private property, and state sovereignty. The striking feature of Lucas's work—and the one that set the tone for subsequent psychiatric commentaries—was that he referred the resolution of political and social questions to what passed for medical knowledge of biology and mental health.[48]

Following Lucas's lead, Emile Renaudin in 1857 and Jacques Moreau de Tours in 1859 drew attention to the way alcoholism left successive generations highly vulnerable to mental and physical stress, resulting in an upswing in the incidence of nervous pathology. Moreau spelled out what this meant for social order. Hereditarily weak individuals, he wrote, could be manipulated by unscrupulous rabblerousers to commit horrendous criminal or political acts.[49] In his 1857 treatise on degeneracy, Morel alerted his countrymen to what he perceived to be the absence of religious sentiment, moral virtue, and sense of duty among the "dangerous" social classes, an absence that he thought had serious consequences for all civilized nations. After years of warning about the danger posed by the degenerate offspring of morally perverse proletarians, Morel felt vindicated when he discovered that 150 children from ages ten to seventeen, most of whom had been caught with firearms behind the Communard barricades, had alcoholic parents or ancestors.[50]

Another psychiatrist who argued that heredity was responsible for antisocial behavior was Ulysée Trélat. His 1861 treatise on lucid madness dealt mainly with its effects on the functioning of family units. However, it also strongly implied that an uninstitutionalized lucid lunatic was not only a curse to his family but also a threat to society. Lucid madmen, Trélat wrote, destroyed family peace because of their irresponsible and erratic actions, which were usually combined with an unsociable nature that made "communal life . . . absolutely impossible." Moreover, because lucid madmen were most often the products of bad heredity themselves, they posed a biological threat to the French state, depriving it by failing to reproduce responsible citizens in future generations. Finally, Trélat emphasized the sinister character of these marginally ill individuals by ascribing to them a special influence over other people that often led to "disaccord" and division within the family and society.[51]

The Paris Commune provided alienists like Morel with data for their hereditarian commentaries on society and politics. Perhaps the clearest example of such a commentary was Dr. J. V. Laborde's *Men and Acts of Insurrection in Paris in Terms of Morbid Psychology: Letters to Dr. Moreau (de Tours)*, published in 1872. As the subtitle indicated, this work was inspired by Moreau's writings; and just as Moreau laid great emphasis on pathological heredity, so Laborde (1830–1903) claimed that heredity was responsible for the criminal and antisocial suggestibility of many Frenchmen,[52] citing Moreau's reference in *Morbid Psychology* to the heightened suggestibility of hereditary neuropaths as a cause of revolutionary mob behavior.[53] Moreau himself praised Laborde's book at the Société on 15 January 1872, when Ludger Lunier also revealed that among the principal Communards there were at least eight certifiable madmen with pronounced bad heredity.[54]

Even when alienists did not specifically cite heredity as responsible for the mental condition of insurrectionists, their accounts of the civil disorder of 1870–1871 could easily be interpreted as hereditarian. For example, Dr. Henri Legrand du Saulle, the assistant physician at the Special Infirmary at the Paris Prefecture of Police, told the Société médico-psychologique on 26 June 1871 that those who lost their senses during political disturbances were not mad because of the emotional impact of the events themselves. He agreed with his colleague C. E. Bourdin that political events were only secondary causes of insanity during periods of civil turmoil.

For one to fall ill because of the political conditions of 1870–1871, Bourdin stated, one had to be predisposed to mental illness. Legrand du Saulle concurred, claiming that

> revolutions and riots only strike the intelligence of predisposed individuals, and only hasten the culmination of a calamity that ought to have been foreseen. An efficient cause quite other than the fall of a throne or a fusillade in the street would have produced identical results. Great social disturbances do not have any disastrous effects on the intellectual faculties of a nation since they are only of a temporary duration.

Legrande du Saulle attributed the apparent cases of insanity produced by "political emotions" to "the great class" of individuals whose minds were "predisposed to morbid lesions." Their minds were predisposed to madness, Legrand du Saulle argued, because they had followed a libertine and morally perverse way of life that had overexcited their passions and depleted their "cerebral energy." Despite his avoidance of hereditarian references, Legrand du Saulle's account was consistent with the theories of hereditarians like Morel, Moreau, and Laborde, who had warned that immoral practices, such as alcoholism and debauchery, could eventually create a hereditary predisposition to insanity and antisocial activity when the political atmosphere grew stressful.[55]

In an 1877 article on the hereditary consequences of alcoholism, Dr. H. Taguet made a more straightforward effort to view the sorry state of France and the political troubles of 1870–1871 from the standpoint of hereditarian and degeneration theory. Taguet, an alienist at the Ville-Evrard asylum, lamented that France's defeat by Germany was directly attributable to its demographic inferiority. Despite the incontestable courage of the French troops, victory belonged to the larger battalions of Prussia, Taguet wrote. The cause of this demographic weakness, he argued, was the atmosphere of "physical and moral decadence" in France, which encouraged the abuse of liquor. Drunkenness affected the nation principally because alcoholics tended to produce offspring that were uncommonly idle, violent, nervous, morally perverse, and, he asserted, highly predisposed to develop suicidal tendencies, epilepsy, deafness, mental retardation, and insanity. Whatever their disability, the progeny of dipsomaniacs were unfit to serve their country, often ending up in the hands of the police and in court.

According to Taguet, they conformed to Morel's theory of degeneracy by producing their own line of offspring that eventually died out and constituted a biological threat to the future of the race and a political liability to the state.[56]

Taguet's article was typical of alienist writing on the social and political problems facing France in the early Third Republic because it blended popular attitudes and interests into a scientific and positivist account that seemed plausible and confirmed conventional morality. In a period of national anxiety over the increasing signs of social dysfunction, demographic weakness, political ineptitude, and moral bankruptcy, psychiatric accounts like Taguet's seemed calculated to minimize these problems by reducing them to emotionally congenial and convincing terms while implying that alienists were alone equipped to deal with them. For example, by maintaining that the trauma of revolutionary events was less important in the etiology of madness during 1870–1871 than the psychological and physical conditions that shaped cerebral predisposition, alienists seemed to ascribe only secondary significance to politics itself. Like good positivists, they argued that the study of the mental characteristics of the population held the key to the discovery of the laws governing politics and the solution to the civil disorder France had experienced since 1789. This form of explanation reassured the public that personal security and private property were threatened far more by the mundane and natural conditions of mental alienation than by sinister Jacobins or communists. It may also have made the insane and the psychologically deviant look more dangerous than they had before, but its medicoscientific patina rendered the specter of revolution and anarchy less traumatic for the middle class. The psychiatrist emerged as a counterrevolutionary public servant whose special knowledge of mental pathology was essential for explaining France's decline.

Some alienists cultivated an image of the psychiatrist as a staunch ally of political order, moral rectitude, and scientific progress. In his account of the turmoil he witnessed at the Prefecture of Police in Paris during the Commune, Legrand du Saulle portrayed himself as a stoic clinician endeavoring to fulfill his medical duties to his patients and civil authority while around him chaos reigned. As he noted, "extreme peril" characterized the situation at the prefecture. The director had been imprisoned. Legrand du Saulle's medical

superior, Charles Lasègue, had been cashiered after twenty years
of service. The chaplain had fled. Eighteen nuns had been expelled.
In addition, "the municipal wheels of government were totally dis-
organized." Amid all this confusion, Legrand du Saulle tried to
maintain his scientific composure and fulfill "the true mandate of a
doctor" by appearing to be unperturbed by the situation. For a
doctor, he declared, "politics does not exist." Physicians were supposed to stand apart from the party infighting, "insurrectionary
plots," and "factious passions" of political life. Legrand du Saulle
echoed the sentiments of the commissioners who had drawn up the
revised statute of the Société médico-psychologique in 1852 when
he suggested that the interests of alienism and the disarray of
revolutionary politics were inimical. The physician, he said, must
"conserve and transmit" medical tradition at all costs and revere
scientific progress above all else.[57] Legrand du Saulle believed
that psychiatry represented clinical enlightenment, intellectual
progress, the continuity of accepted values. His metapolitical
ethos symbolized the attitude of post-1848 French alienism and
demonstrated how far it had distanced itself from its politically radical position during the July Monarchy. Psychiatrists after 1848
characterized themselves as "committed to the prevention of [the]
social conditions of degeneration and aloof from political squab-
bles," disinterested authorities in the moral struggle to restore social discipline and mental health through positivist science.[58]
When French psychiatrists pursued this task using hereditarian
theory, they, like American hereditarians in the same century, offered emotional assurance and intellectual comfort in the face of
phenomena that frightened bourgeois sensibilities and mystified
middle-class ideologues.[59] Psychiatric interpretations of revolution
in general and the hereditary roots of civil disorder in particular
constituted a reassuring myth that "provided comforting resolu-
tions to the anxieties of men of order. It alleviated their guilt and
shame [and] allowed them to project their rage and disgust upon
the 'degenerate' worker."[60] In achieving this result, alienists were
able to strengthen their social position and shift attention away
from the glaring problems plaguing their profession.

The concept of degeneration continued to function successfully
in the 1880s and 1890s as a serviceable medical theory "integrating
the palpable and familiar litany of social pathologies into a discourse
of national decline,"[61] a concrete sign of psychiatry's

sensitivity . . . to the deeper intellectual and cultural currents that affected the entire nation. Pinel's science of moral therapeutics faithfully reflected the rational individualism and the liberal philanthropy of his generation. By the same token, the generation of psychiatry on which Magnan's synthesis put its stamp shared the deep anxieties of its contemporaries about the social effects of hereditary degeneration, the declining birthrate, the "intoxications" of alcohol, drugs, and syphilis, and other mainly biological problems. The shift in concern from the welfare and rehabilitation of the individual to the protection of the family and the social order was a trait that psychiatry had in common with scores of other disciplines and with the French intellectual elite.[62]

Throughout the last two decades of the century, as France's somber mood of despair deepened and its social, political, economic, and demographic problems mounted, psychiatry changed little. It continued to champion a doctrine that promoted the profession by engaging the support of middle class opinion and Third Republic administrators. In an era of Republican "order, social conservatism, and a thorough disapproval of the class antagonisms that had led to the Commune of 1871,"[63] theories of hereditarianism and degeneracy encouraged "minds longing for security"[64] to believe that alienists endorsed a lay Third Republic that would replace religion with "a 'scientific' morality, while preserving the 'natural' structures of the social order." Because leading Republican legislators like Gambetta, Jules Ferry, and Paul Bert "were convinced that political leadership belonged to those schooled in the methods of scientific politics," a psychiatric theory that stressed social solidarity on the basis of biological and organicist truths was a handy weapon for winning the support of politicians whose leader—Gambetta—had sought to curtail the power of psychiatry in the last years of the Second Empire.[65]

Alienist versions of degeneracy theory were anticlerical only in that they weakened public resistance to psychiatry's displacement of the Catholic Church in the institutional treatment of the mad. Otherwise, the hereditarian theory of mental degeneracy did not substantially challenge the idea of human beings as free and self–determining.[66] Morel's original formulation of degeneracy theory in 1857 was blatantly Christian. For him, degeneracy was the deviation from the physical and mental characteristics of Adam and was caused by a host of moral failures and intellectual errors.[67] Morel's theory was consistent with the growing organicist trend in French

mental medicine in the second half of the century, for it conceded
that mental degeneracy was always accompanied by either a functional or a localized structural lesion of the brain, even though this
physical condition could often be traced to emotional states such as
vanity, an antisocial attitude, laziness, or a fondness for liquor.
Morel's emphasis on moral factors in the etiology of mental alienation conformed as well to Catholic sentiments in Third Republic
France. Catholic commentators were "well disposed to degeneracy as an explanation" for the "moral egoism" they felt was destroying modern civilization.[68] Catholics generally seemed to approve
of Morel's reluctance to countenance biological determinism, and
subsequent versions of Morel's ideas did little to erode the notion
of the collective moral responsibility of French policymakers and
savants for the social signs of degeneracy.

Under antipsychiatric public pressure and in conformity with intellectual trends, alienists gradually embraced hereditarianism during the Third Republic. Hereditarianism was primarily a defensive
ideology[69] that enabled alienists to mitigate the professional embarrassment and sociopolitical difficulties stemming from the impasse
in which asylum psychiatry found itself at midcentury. Unsure of its
relationship with the state, uncertain about its medical credentials,
under attack for therapeutic incompetence and evil intentions,
smarting from its keen awareness of its socially marginal status, and
sensitive to criticism by lawyers, clerics, and academic psychologists of its claims to expert knowledge about insanity, alienism embraced a naturalist, biologically oriented, and politically convincing
world view that made it possible to forge an alliance with the
French administrative bureaucracy. The principal asset of hereditarianism was its capacity to depict psychiatrists as politically neutral, orthodox, and uncontroversial, thanks to the growing belief
that science was value-free and objective.[70] As expressed in the
form of degeneracy theory, hereditarianism constituted a plausible
body of secular knowledge regarding the position of men and
women within nature and society, a theory that conformed to the
criteria that defined hegemonic knowledge in a state governed by
men impressed with the ethos of positivist science.[71] Yet hereditarianism in nineteenth-century French psychiatry cannot be understood historically unless viewed as an intellectual response to condi-

tions that alienists believed posed a significant threat to the future of their profession. Anxious about their social status and accessibility to the state's material resources in the years to come, alienists exploited hereditarianism as a way of assuring that they would continue to enjoy institutional and legal prerogatives within French society.

Conclusion

The Social History of Psychiatric Knowledge

Almost as soon as its popularity peaked in the 1890s, the theory of mental degeneracy began to decline. During the heyday of degeneration theory there had never been a shortage of skeptics willing to point out the inconsistencies and imprecision of hereditary degeneracy as a clinical concept, but it was only in the early years of the twentieth century that criticisms of degeneracy theory gained widespread support. When Genil-Perrin observed in 1913 that degeneracy theory was poorly defined, vague, and susceptible to many different psychiatric interpretations, he was saying nothing substantially new.[1] What was new was alienists' growing feeling that degeneracy theory was no longer of much use to them. By 1914 psychiatrists largely agreed with the noted physician Gilbert Ballet (1853–1916), who had written in 1903 that he saw no advantages in including the term *degeneracy* in the twentieth-century psychiatric vocabulary.[2]

There are several likely reasons for the decline of degeneracy theory. Neurologists, principally those of the Charcot school, began experimenting in the 1880s and 1890s with new methods for treating nervous disorders such as hysteria. Serious medical interest in hypnosis at the same time led not only to an increasingly experimental and optimistic attitude toward the cure of certain mental states but also to greater acceptance of the independent reality of an unconscious and dynamic dimension to the mind. The so-called discovery of the unconscious[3] encouraged physicians such as Pierre Janet (1859–1947) to believe that the psychology of the involuntary mind was significant in itself—a belief opposed to degeneracy theory, which held that a patient's mental symptoms, although crucial for classifying mental illnesses, were simply the psychological residues of a diseased and hereditarily tainted nervous system. As these notions grew in popularity among neurologists and other physicians, they challenged psychiatry's customary indifference to the independent significance of mental symptoms, its conventional somaticism, and its faith in theories that rationalized the therapeutic limitations of psychological medicine.

The expansion of neurology around 1900 and its high cultural profile—largely a result of the influence of Charcot—had the effect of discrediting alienism's traditional assumptions and compelling it to reassess its relationship to both the asylum and the asylum's institutionalized population. Psychiatry and neurology began to merge as the century came to a close, a process that tended to weaken alienist attachments to the asylum. It was no coincidence that Gilbert Ballet, one of the most persuasive critics of Magnan's degeneracy theory, was also a leader in the campaign for rapprochement between alienists and neurologists early in the new century.[4] With its greater scientific prestige, a product mainly of its roots in organic medicine, neurology reminded alienists that hospital psychiatry remained isolated from the rest of organized medicine as long as its primary locus was the asylum.

The psychiatric reassessment of the asylum was accelerated by developing distinctions between insanity and mental illness. In France, as in California, it was believed that many of those who previously might have been classified as insane were only mildly disturbed and could be cured without confinement.[5] This meant that isolation in an asylum was no longer the only way to treat psychologically disturbed persons and that the therapeutic domain of psychiatry extended beyond the walls of the asylum. Similarly, the growth of the mental hygiene movement and the many examples of "war neuroses" between 1914 and 1918 fostered the notion that otherwise normal individuals could easily become mentally disturbed. This further encouraged psychiatrists to reevaluate their relationship to their traditional patients, particularly because there now existed potential clients who were more affluent and socially respectable on the whole than the destitute and often violent inmates of the typical nineteenth-century asylum.[6]

The psychiatric willingness to look beyond the asylum for more promising therapeutic horizons signaled the end of "alienism" and the beginning of "psychiatry." It also sounded the death knell of degeneracy theory, which was tied indissolubly to the fortunes of the nineteenth-century asylum in France. The asylum had become by the end of the nineteenth century a place of confinement and detention for a population that was considered to be highly resistant to treatment and cure largely because of hereditary disease. As one psychiatrist complained in 1913, the organization and hierarchy of a typical late nineteenth-century asylum were designed to facilitate the surveillance and clinical observation of patients. The result, he argued, was that alienists had treated only the patients' symptoms and not the cause of mental illness. This is precisely what Morel had lamented fifty years earlier. The critical difference between Morel and his early twentieth-century successors was that the latter were willing to reform the services offered by mental hospitals; for example, adding outpatient wards for the treatment of psychoneuroses. Without these changes, psychiatrists feared, curable patients would seek treatment at nonpsychiatric hospitals, reinforcing the image of the mental hospital as an institution for the long-term incarceration of incurable persons. "I believe it is indispensable," a psychiatrist wrote in 1913, "to make the asylum a true place for improving health (*une véritable maison de santé*)."[7] When psychiatrists concluded that their identification with the custodial public asylum had become a liability, the fortunes of degeneracy theory suffered because one of the theory's principal advantages to alienists had been its capacity to justify the existence of the asylum and the asylum physician's claims to expertise.

The growing sense of "nationalist revival" and regeneration in France, especially after the Tangiers crisis of 1905, further undermined psychiatric and broader cultural attachment to ideas of degeneration. While reliance on the discourse of degeneration did not cease in the decade leading up to World War I, there were increasing calls for a rejection of nihilism and pessimism in matters of national health and fitness. Military preparedness for the anticipated clash with Imperial Germany had much to do with this revival of confidence and will, but widespread interest in sport and physical culture also contributed to it. Physicians gradually stopped believing that degeneration was an irreversible process and grew optimistic about the possibilities of treating even the more severe forms of degeneracy, such as mental retardation. The emergence of a French eugenics movement in the early twentieth century reinforced medical convictions that something positive could be done to produce stronger and healthier French men and women.[8]

The decline of degeneracy theory may also be attributable to the emergence in the 1890s of a new social doctrine called *solidarism*. Solidarism was a reaction to the political crises and economic difficulties of the 1880s. By 1890 it was clear that the political left and right had rejected the "opportunist" Third Republic ushered in after Marshall MacMahon's resignation in 1877. Opportunist republicans like Léon Gambetta, Paul Bert, and Jules Ferry had tended to propose educational solutions to social problems such as labor unrest and class friction. They believed that secular education was the key to ending the ignorance of the masses; ignorance, they thought, was the primary cause of the lower classes' attraction to slogans and symbols that stressed social conflict.[9] Solidarism endorsed a more activist social program of welfare for the poor and working classes than the one favored by the Opportunists. By the turn of the century, republican governments had largely dispensed with laissez-faire approaches to social problems, passing a flood of social welfare legislation and emphasizing instead the founding of mutual benefit societies designed to provide a range of social services for the masses.[10] This new social philosophy went far beyond the Opportunist and positivist emphasis on moral education according to the principles of natural science, an ethos that lay at the heart of asylum practice and theory. The late nineteenth-century asylum was perceived as a primarily secular institution in which the alienist used his moral probity and scientific training to encourage patients to disavow their antisocial ideas and perverse sentiments. The moral treatment used by the asylum physician stood as an example of the way in which the methods of natural science could be exploited to improve the morality of the masses by fostering self-reliance and positive attitudes toward work. It showed, in short, how education could be both moral and scientific at the same time. Confining lunatics in public institutions for moral and pedagogical purposes became less justifiable when the Opportunist notion of secular education as the principal weapon for destroying the ignorance and selfishness of the pauper classes fell out of favor.

The French state's increasing assistance to the poor probably also influenced attitudes toward the asylum. The redeployment of state resources into alternative welfare programs doubtless undermined bureaucratic commitment to the asylum as a catchall form of public assistance, reinforcing the persistent opinion that asylums were expensive institutions to maintain. While the early twentieth century did not witness anything close to the decarceration movement of the 1960s and 1970s, it is arguable that the social legislation passed by republican governments in the years leading up to World War I had an effect on the mental hospital similar to that exerted by the expansion of welfare services in the United States and England since the 1950s: commitment to the asylum declined when it was realized that there were other programs for controlling deviant behavior and discouraging dissent.[11] Psychiatrists, sensing that the asylum was losing its primacy as an institutional form of public assistance, began in the new century to consider other ways of dealing with mental illness.

Doubtless, too, the discovery in 1913 of the organism responsible for syphilis in the brain of paretic sufferers, which showed that general paresis was the tertiary stage of syphilis, not a hereditary affliction as many French physicians believed in the 1880s, increased medical impatience with hereditary degeneracy theory. Although this development could have contributed to the fall of degeneracy theory, it is important to note that degeneracy theory had thrived in the first place not because it was supported by a wealth of empirical evidence but because it justified the professional practices of alienism during a period when psychological medicine was undergoing a barrage of criticism from a variety of social, political, and cultural groups. It was the shifting professional circumstances that shaped the fate of degeneracy theory, not the acknowledgment of its anomalies or its inconsistency with new biomedical discoveries. In fact, as I have argued elsewhere,[12] psychiatry as a profession may be in a perpetual state of Kuhnian crisis by virtue of its inherent cognitive and empirical difficulties.[13] As a result, psychiatric knowledge has a fluid character that—combined with the fact that it never ceases to be free of "social" considerations—virtually guarantees that it will be a shifting blend of cultural attitudes, social values, political beliefs, and professional imperatives. The task for the historian is to unravel the complex process of theory formation in psychological medicine and trace the causal paths linking society, state, profession, and knowledge.

The correspondence between professionalization and psychiatric ideas in nineteenth-century France takes on added meaning when viewed in relation to nineteenth-century Anglo-American alienism. While the chronology was not everywhere the same, France, Britain, the United States, and Canada witnessed the same "morphology of reform." The beginning of the nineteenth century saw innovative attempts to cure mental illness through institutionalization and individual moral treatment. Whether lay or medical, reformers tended to bring a missionary zeal to the task of curing their patients. They distrusted customary medical therapies, abhorred the brutality of earlier methods of treatment, and were optimistic that mental disease could be cured when the patient's emotional needs were addressed properly.

After midcentury this optimism faded. The treatment of mental illness was entrusted primarily to licensed physicians, and the claim of talented amateurs to therapeutic skill increasingly rang hollow. At the same time families and civil authorities began to exploit the new asylums by committing senile, severely handicapped, or troublesome persons, a policy that led to institutional overcrowding and a disproportionate number of incurable cases. The irony is that the public, although willing to patronize modern asylums, did not value hospital psychiatry highly and often turned against asylum physicians when suspicions of unfair confinement arose in the 1860s and 1870s. When asylums became "factories of incurability" largely populated by paupers, "humane treatment, flexibility, personal attention, and sophisticated reflection" ceased to characterize asylum practice.[14] Hereditarian explanations grew popular as asylum conditions deteriorated near the end of the century because they rationalized medicine's inability to surmount the therapeutic difficulties of hospital psychiatry. Hereditarianism endorsed the notion that asylums were full of pauper lunatics whose incurability derived from their hereditary weaknesses and their unwillingness to desist from depraved and unhealthy activities. Hereditarian explanations like degeneracy theory held that there was a physiological reason for the therapeutic futility of asylum physicians, that the poor were morally responsible for their mental maladies, and that they therefore needed to be confined in institutions whose administrative structures held out the only hope for rehabilitation.

Aspects of this striking pattern in the social history of knowledge have been identified by many historians of Anglo-American psychiatry. One aspect identified in most of their accounts, and one that has occupied center stage here, is the vulnerable status of the nineteenth-century alienist. Even in France, where alienists enjoyed the unprecedented professional privileges accorded to medicine by Napoleon in 1803, psychiatry faced strong opposition to its claims to exclusive therapeutic and diagnostic prerogatives in the management of insanity. French psychiatrists shared with their Anglo-American colleagues the complaint that the state rarely subsidized asylums sufficiently to accommodate the growing inmate populations. Governments may have valued the penal functions performed by asylum physicians, but they did not always show their appreciation in the form of material support. Similarly, if governments did not bow in the end to the critics of alienism who called for deinstitutionalization policies and the reduction of psychiatric legal powers, they were never very vocal in their support of psychiatry. French alienists had to deal with an antipsychiatric campaign that appears to have been more sustained and serious than the "lunacy panics" in England[15] or the attacks on U.S. asylum superintendents in post-Civil War newspapers and trials.[16] Unlike the situation in late imperial Russia,[17] French calls for the deinstitutionalization of psychiatry in the 1860s did not attract elite support, and therein lies the reason for the failure of the antipsychiatric movement. But there is no discounting the psychiatric fear in the 1860s that elite support *might* swing behind the proponents of deinstitutionalization and rob alienists of their asylum powers.

A historical explanation of psychiatric theory must take into account these defensive features of mental medicine. Since the origins of the modern asylum at the beginning of the nineteenth century, psychiatrists have had to rationalize the political fact that their specialty status was attained before they possessed a rigorously exact body of knowledge on which to base it. Moreover, because psychiatrists claim both professional expertise and membership in general medicine, they have found it harder than, say, nursing and social work to explain how they possess expertise in the treatment of mental and nervous disease.[18] As physicians, psychiatrists are often hard-pressed to meet the standards of expertise set by other medical specialties such as bacteriology, physiology, or surgery. This vulnerability to criticism may explain why psychiatrists have been "nevertheless quite resourceful and effective in defending" their status and prerogatives.[19] Simply put, psychiatrists have had to be resourceful and experimentally innovative, if only to demonstrate that as physicians they were entitled exclusively to treat the mentally ill. In therapeutic matters, this has led to some regrettable developments.[20] In terms of psychiatric theory, it has led to some inventive use of what passed for contemporaneous science, largely in order to reinforce psychiatry's cultural authority as well as to mystify mental health and encourage laypersons to defer to medical opinion.

The restoration through science of mental health's legitimate complexity[21] differed somewhat from one country to the next. For example, for most of the nineteenth century, psychiatric interest in medical science was much greater in France than it was in the United States, where asylum superintendents tended to stress their expertise in practical matters such as asylum design, construction, and management rather than their knowledge of insanity's nature and pathology.[22] However, once the combined criticism of neurologists, civil libertarians, and social administrators produced a "crisis of professional legitimacy" for psychiatry from 1881 to 1885, medical superintendents in the United States began expressing an interest in the more scientific dimensions of mental disease, such as pathology, physiology, and pharmacology.[23] In doing so, they resembled their French colleagues, who two decades earlier had constructed an ideological framework that justified their practice, role, and status and "incorporate[d] general norms and values."[24] This ideological framework—hereditary degeneracy—seems on one level to have had as little relevance to psychiatric practice in mental hospitals as did twentieth-century Freudian concepts.[25] The same could be said for Morel's and Magnan's ideas: while lip service was paid to their concepts of disease in the second half of the nineteenth century, the concepts did little to change a therapeutic tradition based on the alleged efficacy of drugs and the moral authority of the asylum physician. They are valuable to the historian of psychiatry because, like many explanations of disease,

they "tell . . . us more about individuals and the groups they rep-
resent than about the nature of disease," and because they suggest
where psychiatry's professional interests lay at specific points in its
history.[26]

The picture drawn here of psychiatry is both indebted to and
critical of Michel Foucault's description of the relations between
professional knowledge and the hegemony of the "disciplines" in
modern western society. Foucault was right to stress the extent to
which the growth of the professions in the last two centuries is due
to the evolution of bodies of knowledge that authorize the widening
of state power and control over the "docile bodies" of disadvantaged
social groups. For example, psychiatrists have consistently tried to
encourage legislators and the public to believe that there were far
more insane persons and dangerous lunatics than any nonphysician
could imagine or treat and, until recently, that they should be confined for their own good and that of society. At the same time, there
is a seamless quality to Foucault's model that, like many sociological
models, fits historical reality poorly. This is most evident in the way
Foucault has largely ignored how physicians gained control of asylums or the recurrent bouts of frustration and anxiety that have
characterized psychiatry to the present day. His one-dimensional
view of psychiatry as a profession boldly carving out new territories
for exploitation (or psychiatric "imperialism" as it has been called)
has to be tempered by the realization that its fortunes have waxed
and waned as opposition has from time to time threatened to undo
much of what psychiatrists have managed to achieve since Pinel's
days. Degeneracy theory, as Daniel Pick has shown, exemplified
both the "imperialistic" and the vulnerable features of psychiatry's
professionalization in the nineteenth century. Degeneration was
first and foremost a reflection of psychiatry's preoccupation with its
own interests, but those interests had as much to do with preserving power as with extending power.[27]

It is instructive to reflect on this chapter in psychiatry's past at a
time when psychological medicine is still undergoing a "crisis of
legitimacy."[28] Today there is much talk about the genetic roots of
schizophrenia and the failure of deinstitutionalization as a social
policy, just as there was a great deal of debate in France after 1850
about the effectiveness of forms of public assistance to the insane
other than the asylum. Then, as now, many psychiatrists were

highly critical of noninstitutional treatment—particularly for those psychotics prone to violence—and publicly expressed their confidence that the extent to which heredity influenced the incidence of mental illness could be determined. It is also worth noting that in both instances the trend toward hereditarian explanations of mental illness followed on the heels of widespread antipsychiatric movements that questioned the right of psychiatry to claim exclusive knowledge of insanity's diagnosis and treatment. Whereas nineteenth-century French psychiatrists had to struggle to reduce the role of the clerical orders in the institutional care of the insane, psychiatrists in the 1990s must deal with intensifying interprofessional competition from nonmedical workers in mental health care.[29] If today we are witnessing, as some contend, a psychiatric return to neurobiological and genetic explanations of deviant affective and behavioral phenomena, it is well to remember how a similar trend in late nineteenth-century French psychiatry developed. In France the asylum largely changed from a center for rehabilitation and benevolent care to an institution for the confinement, detention, and discipline of persons considered to be dangerous to themselves and to social order by virtue of their hereditary taint. Will there be a corresponding resurgence of the mental hospital's penal functions now that more psychiatrists and public officials are publicizing the danger posed by psychotics who roam the streets under the community services system?[30] Will limits be placed on the legal rights of mental patients to refuse medical treatment? Public decisions taken at transitional stages in the history of social policy toward the mentally ill have had consequences that shaped cultural attitudes toward the very structure and relations of power in Western society.[31] With a growing historical awareness of the role the liberal professions, including medicine, have played in Western society, the public is now in a position to determine to what extent these occupational groups in fact enjoy privileged access to special knowledge and exclusive competence in certain spheres of social practice. This is the critical first step toward identifying the historical organization of power and consent in Western culture.

Notes

Introduction

1. Théophile Roussel, *Notes et documents concernant la législation française et les législations étrangères sur les aliénés. Annexe au procès-verbal de la séance du 20 mai 1884. Commission relative à la révision de la loi du 30 juin 1838 sur les aliénés*, 2 vols. (Paris: P. Mouillot, 1884), 1:298.

2. James T. Patterson, *The Dread Disease: Cancer and Modern American Culture* (Cambridge: Harvard University Press, 1987).

3. Georges Genil-Perrin, *Histoire des origines et de l'évolution de l'idée de dégénérescence en médecine mentale* (Paris: Leclerc, 1913), p. 9.

4. For confirmation of this tendency to equate degeneracy and heredity, see Laurent Cerise's remarks at the meeting of the Société médico-psychologique on 29 June 1857, *Annales médico-psychologiques* 3 (1857):627.

5. Genil-Perrin, *Histoire*, pp. 11–12.

6. Other treatments of degeneracy theory include François Bing, "La Théorie de la dégénérescence," in Jacques Postel and Claude Quétel, eds., *Nouvelle histoire de la psychiatrie* (Toulouse: Privat, 1983), pp. 351–64; Peter Burgener, *Die Einflüsse des Zeitgenössischen Denkens in Morels Begriff der "Dégénérescence"* (Zurich: Juris-Verlag, 1964); Jean Borie, *Mythologies de l'hérédité au XIXe siècle* (Paris: Editions galilées, 1981); Robert Castel, *L'Ordre psychiatrique: L'Âge d'or de l'aliénisme* (Paris: Editions de Minuit, 1976); Ruth Friedlander, "B. A. Morel and the Theory of Degenerescence: The Introduction of Anthropology into Psychiatry" (Ph.D. diss., University of California at San Francisco, 1973); Milton

Gold, "The Early Psychiatrists on Degeneracy and Genius," *Psychoanalysis and the Psychoanalytic Review* 47 (1960–61):37–55. The most recent and authoritative account of degeneration is Daniel Pick's *Faces of Degeneration: A European Disorder, c.1848–c.1918* (Cambridge: Cambridge University Press, 1989).

7. Richard Hunter and Ida MacAlpine, eds., *Three Hundred Years of Psychiatry, 1535–1860* (London: Oxford University Press, 1963), p. vii.

8. John Romano, "American Psychiatry: Past, Present, and Future," in G. Kriegman, R. D. Gardner, and D. W. Abse, eds., *American Psychiatry: Past, Present, and Future* (Charlottesville: University Press of Virginia, 1975), p. 29.

9. Michel Foucault, *Madness and Civilization: A History of Insanity in the Age of Reason,* trans. Richard Howard (New York: Random House, 1965), pp. 38–64.

10. Colin Jones, "The Treatment of the Insane in Eighteenth- and Early Nineteenth-Century Montpellier: A Contribution to the Prehistory of the Lunatic Asylum in Provincial France," *Medical History* 24 (1980):371–90.

11. For the wish that modern American psychiatrists develop such a concept, see Romano, "American Psychiatry," pp. 28–44.

12. Roger Cooter, "Phrenology and British Alienists ca. 1825–1845," in Andrew Scull, ed., *Madhouses, Mad-Doctors, and Madmen: The Social History of Psychiatry in the Victorian Era* (Philadelphia: Univ. of Pennsylvania Press, 1981), p. 58. See also his *The Cultural Meaning of Popular Science: Phrenology and the Organization of Consent in Nineteenth-Century Britain* (Cambridge: Cambridge University Press, 1984).

13. Charles Rosenberg, *No Other Gods: On Science and American Social Thought* (Baltimore: Johns Hopkins University Press, 1976). See chap. 1, "The Bitter Fruit: Heredity, Disease, and Social Thought in Nineteenth-Century America," p. 53.

14. See Paul Forman, "Weimar Culture, Causality, and Quantum Theory, 1918–1927: Adaptation by German Physicists and Mathematicians to a Hostile Intellectual Environment," *Historical Studies in the Physical Sciences* 3 (1971):1–115; see also Theodore M. Brown, "The College of Physicians and the Acceptance of Iatromechanism in England, 1665–1695," *Bulletin of the History of Medicine,* 44 (1970):12–30.

15. For confirmation of this conclusion, see Castel, *L'Ordre Psychiatrique,* p. 271n6. See also Antoine Ritti, *Histoire des travaux de la Société médico-psychologique et éloges de ses membres,* 2 vols. (Paris: Masson, 1913–1914).

16. One exception is Jan Goldstein's account of the "Esquirol Circle" in her "French Psychiatry in Social and Political Context: The Formation

of a New Profession, 1820–1860" (Ph.D. diss., Columbia University, 1978). See also her *Console and Classify: The French Psychiatric Profession in the Nineteenth Century* (Cambridge: Cambridge University Press, 1987).

17. Kenneth L. Caneva, "What Should We Do with the Monster? Electromagnetism and the Psychosociology of Knowledge," in Everett Mendelsohn and Yehuda Elkana, eds., *Sciences and Cultures: Sociology of the Sciences* 5 (1981):103.

18. For a recent collection of essays on the relations between the liberal professions and the French state from 1700 to 1900, see Gerald L. Geison, ed., *Professions and the French State, 1700–1900* (Philadelphia: Univ. of Pennsylvania Press, 1984). See also Burton J. Bledstein, *The Culture of Professionalism: The Middle Class and the Development of Higher Education in America* (New York: Norton, 1976). For an astute discussion of the advantages and disadvantages of using the term *professionalization* to describe the experience of French medicine in the nineteenth century, see Matthew Ramsey, *Professional and Popular Medicine in France, 1770–1830: The Social World of Medical Practice* (Cambridge: Cambridge University Press, 1988), pp. 1–5.

19. S. E. D. Shortt, "Physicians, Science, and Status: Issues in the Professionalization of Anglo-American Medicine in the Nineteenth Century," *Medical History* 27 (1983):52.

20. George D. Sussman, "The Glut of Doctors in Nineteenth-Century France," *Comparative Studies in Society and History* 19 (1977):287.

21. George Weisz, "The Politics of Medical Professionalization in France, 1845–1848," *Journal of Social History* 12 (1978):23.

22. Shortt, "Physicians, Science, and Status," p. 62; for a more detailed historical study of "marginal men" and the rhetoric of science, see Arnold Thackray, "Natural Knowledge in Cultural Context: The Manchester Model," *American Historical Review* 79 (1974):672–709.

23. See Robert A. Nye, *Crime, Madness, and Politics in Modern France: The Medical Concept of National Decline* (Princeton: Princeton University Press, 1984).

24. For parallel developments in nineteenth-century British psychiatry, see L. S. Jacyna, "Somatic Theories of Mind and the Interests of Medicine in Britain, 1850–1879," *Medical History* 26 (1982):253–54.

25. S. E. D. Shortt, *Victorian Lunacy: Richard M. Bucke and the Practice of Late Nineteenth-Century Psychiatry* (Cambridge: Cambridge University Press, 1986), p. 108.

26. William F. Bynum, "Rationales for Therapy in British Psychiatry, 1780–1835," in Scull, *Madhouses*, p. 52.

27. Goldstein, *Console and Classify*, p. 379.

Chapter One:
The State of Psychiatric Practice and
Knowledge in the Nineteenth Century

1. Matthew Ramsey, "The Politics of Professional Monopoly in Nineteenth–Century Medicine: The French Model and its Rivals," in Gerald L. Geison, ed., *Professions and the French State, 1700–1900* (Philadelphia: Univ. of Pennsylvania Press, 1984), p. 240.

2. George Weisz, "The Politics of Medical Professionalization in France, 1845–1848," *Journal of Social History*, 12 (1978):3–30, especially p. 13.

3. Lenore O'Boyle, "The Middle Class in Western Europe, 1815–1848," *American Historical Review* 71 (1966):826–45.

4. Edouard Charton, *Dictionnaire des professions*, 2nd ed. (Paris: V. Lenoremant, 1851), pp. 389–90. Cited in Weisz, "Politics of Medical Professionalization," p. 7.

5. Erwin H. Ackerknecht, *Medicine at the Paris Hospital, 1794–1848* (Baltimore: Johns Hopkins University Press, 1967), pp. 185–86.

6. Jacques Léonard, "Les Guérisseurs en France au XIXe siècle," *Revue d'histoire moderne et contemporaine* 27 (1980):515. For an example of psychiatric and medical disagreement over the therapeutic value of mesmerism and hypnotism, see the debates at the Société médico-psychologique in 1857–1858 in *Annales médico-psychologiques* 3 (1857): 601–619, 630–635; 4 (1858):228–235, 240–249, 258–265, 312–324 (hereafter cited as *Amp*.).

7. Matthew Ramsey, "Medical Power and Popular Medicine: Illegal Healers in Nineteenth-Century France," *Journal of Social History* 10 (1977):560–87.

8. Léonard, "Les Guérisseurs," p. 505.

9. See the report of the *Lancet*'s special Paris correspondent, *Lancet* 2 (1861):261.

10. Ramsey, "Politics of Professional Monopoly," p. 228.

11. Weisz, "Politics of Medical Professionalization," p. 23.

12. Ramsey, "Politics of Professional Monopoly," p. 229.

13. Weisz, "Politics of Medical Professionalization," p. 8.

14. Jan Ellen Goldstein, "French Psychiatry in Social and Political Context: The Formation of a New Profession, 1820–1860" (Ph.D. diss., Columbia University, 1978), pp. 303, 315.

15. J. Baillarger, "Association des médecins des hospices d'aliénés en Angleterre. De l'utilité que pourrait avoir une association semblable parmi les médecins français," *Amp.* 1 (1843):181–83.

16. Cl. Michéa, "Lettre au citoyen Thierry, directeur des hôpitaux et

hospices civils de Paris, sur l'injustice et le danger qu'il y aurait à supprimer le concours spécial pour les places de médecine des aliénés," *Amp*. 11 (1848):451–53.

17. George D. Sussman, "The Glut of Doctors in Nineteenth-Century France," *Comparative Studies in Society and History* 19 (1977): 287–304.

18. For French psychiatry's adoption of the monomania defence in legal medicine, see Jan Goldstein, *Console and Classify: The French Psychiatric Profession in the Nineteenth Century* (Cambridge: Cambridge University Press, 1987), chap. 5. See also Ruth Harris, *Murders and Madness: Medicine, Law, and Society in the Fin-de-Siècle* (Oxford: Oxford University Press, 1989), especially chaps. 2 and 3.

19. See Colin Jones, "The Treatment of the Insane in Eighteenth- and Early Nineteenth-Century Montpellier: A Contribution to the Prehistory of the Lunatic Asylum in Provincial France," *Medical History* 24 (1980):371–90.

20. Quoted in Gerard Bleandonu and Guy Le Gaufey, "The Creation of the Insane Asylums of Auxerre and Paris," in Robert Forster and Orest Ranum, eds., *Deviants and the Abandoned in French Society*, trans. Elborg Forster and Patrick M. Ranum, 7 vols. (Baltimore: Johns Hopkins University Press, 1978), 4:188–89.

21. Jones, "Treatment of the Insane," pp. 371–72.

22. H. Girard de Cailleux, "Considérations générales sur l'ensemble du service des aliénés du département de la Seine," *Amp*. 7 (1861):267–68. See also H. Legrand du Saulle's review of Dr. Berthier's *Excursions scientifiques dans les asiles d'aliénés* in *Amp*. 3 (1864):453–55.

23. *Amp*. 1 (1869):283.

24. 27 Dec. 1852 meeting of the Société médico-psychologique, *Amp*. 5 (1853):325.

25. 26 Dec. 1864 meeting of the Société médico-psychologique, *Amp*. 5 (1865):290–91.

26. For the text of the 1838 law, see Robert Castel, *L'Ordre psychiatrique: L'Âge d'or de l'aliénisme* (Paris: Editions de Minuit, 1976), pp. 316–24.

27. Augustin Constans, Ludger Lunier, and Edouard Jean-Baptiste Dumesnil, *Rapport générale à M. le Ministre de l'Intérieur sur le service des aliénés en 1874* (Paris: Imprimerie nationale, 1878), p. 47 (hereafter cited as CLD, *Rapport*).

28. Ibid., p. 54.

29. For the living conditions and demographic makeup of Paris in the first half of the nineteenth century, see Louis Chevalier, *Labouring Classes and Dangerous Classes in Paris during the First Half of the Nine-*

teenth Century, trans. Frank Jellinek (New York: Howard Fertig, 1973). See also Mark Daniel Alexander, "The Administration of Madness and Attitudes Towards the Insane in Nineteenth-Century Paris" (Ph.D. diss., Johns Hopkins University, 1976).

30. CLD, *Rapport*, p. 61.

31. Georges Lanteri-Laura, "Chronicité dans la psychiatrie française moderne," *Annales E.S.C.* 27 (1972):548–68.

32. CLD, *Rapport*, p. 66.

33. Ibid., p. 478.

34. Ibid., pp. 552–53.

35. A. Planés, "Mouvement de l'aliénation mentale à Paris (1872–1885)," *Amp*. 5 (1887):60–70, 229–53.

36. CLD, *Rapport*, pp. 552–53.

37. Ibid.

38. *Amp*. 1 (1849):427.

39. Planés, "Mouvement de l'aliénation mentale à Paris (1872–1885)," p. 236.

40. "Chronique," *Amp*. 8 (1888):8.

41. L. Lunier, "Du mouvement de l'aliénation mentale en France de 1835 à 1882," *Amp*. 12 (1884):205.

42. Ibid., pp. 206–7.

43. Ibid., p. 206.

44. For example, see the comments of Dr. Archambault in his review of J.-B. Cazauvielh's *Du suicide, de l'aliénation mentale, et des crimes contre les personnes* in *Amp*. 1 (1843):170.

45. Léonard, "Les Guérisseurs," p. 505.

46. Erwin H. Ackerknecht, *A Short History of Psychiatry*, trans. Sula Wolff (New York: Hafner, 1965), p. viii. See also Roger Smith, *Trial by Medicine: Insanity and Responsibility in Victorian Trials* (Edinburgh: Edinburgh University Press, 1981), pp. 6–7 for a description of the stigma borne by British alienists during the Victorian era.

47. Dr. Hospital, "Le Martyrologie de la psychiatrie," *Amp*. 6 (1887):353–54. Author's emphasis.

48. Castel, *L'Ordre psychiatrique*, pp. 234–35.

49. CLD, *Rapport*, pp. 54–62.

50. Goldstein has argued that in fact the government of the July Monarchy paid a great deal of attention to the way in which the asylum law functioned after 1838. Goldstein, *Console and Classify*, p. 307n. For a dissenting view, see Castel, *L'Ordre psychiatrique*, pp. 235, 241–43.

51. CLD, *Rapport*, p. 52.

52. Alexandre Brierre de Boismont, "Observations sur le nouveau

mode de nomination des médecins d'asiles d'aliénés," *L'union médicale,* 27 April 1852.

53. CLD, *Rapport,* pp. 56, 161, 487.

54. Goldstein, *Console and Classify,* p. 307. See also chap. 6, pp. 198, 217, 307–21.

55. Auguste Motet, review of A. Voisin's *Leçons cliniques sur les maladies mentales* in *Amp.* 16 (1876):312–15. See also A. Linas, *Le passé, le présent, et l'avenir de la médecine mentale en France* (Paris: Masson, 1863), p. 3.

56. Jean-Pierre Falret, "De l'enseignement clinique des maladies mentales," *Amp.* 1 (1849):524–79. For a detailed account of resistance to clinical instruction in psychiatry, see Goldstein, *Console and Classify,* pp. 345–50.

57. Jules Falret, Introduction to his translation of W. Griesinger's "La Pathologie mentale au point de vue de l'école somatique allemande," *Amp.* 5 (1865):4.

58. B. A. Morel, *Traité des dégénérescences physiques, intellectuelles, et morales de l'espèce humaine* (Paris: Baillière, 1857), p. xii.

59. For the authoritative account of Parisian medicine in the early nineteenth century, see Ackerknecht, *Medicine at the Paris Hospital.*

60. L. Delasiauve, review of L. F. Calmeil's *Traité des maladies inflammatoires du cerveau* in *Amp.* 6 (1860):473.

61. For Pinel's comments on pathological anatomy, see Philippe Pinel, *A Treatise on Insanity,* trans. D. D. Davis (Sheffield: Cadell and Davies, 1806; reprint, New York: Hafner, 1962), pp. 110–11; 131–33.

62. J. E. D. Esquirol, *Mental Maladies: A Treatise on Insanity,* trans. E. K. Hunt (Philadelphia: Lea and Blanchard, 1845), pp. 396–97.

63. U. Trélat, "De la paralysie générale," *Amp.* 1 (1855):240.

64. A. Brierre de Boismont, *Hallucinations: Or, the Rational History of Apparitions, Visions, Dreams, Ecstasy, Magnetism, and Somnambulism,* 1st American ed. from 2nd enlarged French ed. (Philadelphia: Lindsay and Blackiston, 1853), p. 28.

65. Robert M. Young, *Mind, Brain, and Adaptation in the Nineteenth Century: Cerebral Localization and its Biological Context from Gall to Ferrier* (Oxford: Clarendon Press, 1970), p. 56.

66. J. P. Falret, *Maladies mentales et des asiles d'aliénés* (Paris: Baillière, 1864), pp. v–vi; Georges Lanteri-Laura, *Histoire de la phrenologie* (Paris: Presses universitaires de France, 1970), pp. 158–59. See also Angus McLaren, "A Prehistory of the Social Sciences: Phrenology in France," *Comparative Studies in Society and History* 23 (1981):3–22.

67. Ach. Foville, "Des relations entre les troubles de la motilité

dans la paralysie générale et les lésions de la couche corticale des circonvolutions fronto-pariétales," *Amp* 17 (1877):5–6. See also Young, *Mind, Brain and Adaptation*, pp. 55–74.

68. CLD, *Rapport*, p. i.

69. Cited in A. Linas, review of L. Marcé's *Traité pratique des maladies mentales* in *Amp*. 1 (1863):298.

70. L. Peisse, *La Médecine et les médecins: philosophie, doctrines, institutions, critiques, moeurs, et biographies médicales*, 2 vols. (Paris: Baillière, 1857) 2:19–22.

71. John Charles Bucknill and Daniel H. Tuke, *A Manual of Psychological Medicine* (Philadelphia, 1858; reprint, New York: Hafner, 1968), p. 341.

72. Ibid., p. 342.

73. 25 Feb. 1856 meeting of the Société medico-psychologique, *Amp*. 2 (1856):391–93.

74. For an account of Griesinger and his career, see Otto Marx, "Wilhelm Griesinger and the History of Psychiatry: A Reassessment," *Bulletin of the History of Medicine* 46 (1972):519–44.

75. W. Griesinger, *Mental Pathology and Therapeutics*, trans. C. Lockhart Robertson and James Rutherford (London: 1867; reprint, New York: Hafner, 1965), pp. 6–8.

76. J. P. Falret, *Maladies mentales*, p. xxv.

77. J. Falret, Introduction to Griesinger's "La pathologie mentale", p. 4.

78. Griesinger, *Mental Pathology and Therapeutics*, p. 9.

79. Bucknill and Tuke, *A Manual of Psychological Medicine*, p. 267.

80. A. Brierre de Boismont, *Hallucinations*, p. ix.

81. For example, see A. Linas, review of J. P. Falret's *Des maladies mentales et des asiles d'aliénés* in *Amp*. 5 (1865):359.

82. L. F. E. Renaudin, *Etudes médico-psychologiques sur l'aliénation mentale* (Paris: Baillière, 1854), p. 9.

83. 12 Nov. 1860 meeting of the Société médico-psychologique, *Amp*. 7 (1861):131.

84. 26 Nov. 1860 meeting of the Société, Ibid., pp. 172–73.

85. 25 Feb. 1861 meeting of the Société, Ibid., pp. 459–60.

86. Ibid., pp. 463–64.

87. W. Griesinger, *Traité des maladies mentales, pathologie et thérapeutique*, trans. of 2nd German ed., 1861, by Dr. Doumic with notes by J. Baillarger (Paris: Delahaye, 1865), pp. 155–56n.

88. J. Moreau de Tours, *Hashish and Mental Illness*, ed. Helene Peters and Gabriel G. Nahas, trans. of 1845 ed. by Gordon J. Barnett (New York: Raven Press, 1973), p. 135.

89. Griesinger, *Traité*, p. 5n.

90. 25 Feb. 1861 meeting of the Société médico-psychologique, *Amp.* 7 (1861):466–67.

91. Ch. Lasègue, review of Moreau's *Du haschisch et de l'aliénation mentale* in *Amp.* 7 (1846):459–63.

92. Gerald N. Grob, "Rediscovering Asylums: The Unhistorical History of the Mental Hospital," in Morris J. Vogel and Charles E. Rosenberg, eds., *The Therapeutic Revolution: Essays in the Social History of American Medicine* (Philadelphia: University of Pennsylvania Press, 1979), p. 141.

93. Peisse, *La Médecine*, 2:11.

94. J. B. E. Bousquet, 8 May 1855 meeting of the Imperial Academy of Medicine, reprinted in *Amp.* 1 (1855):451.

95. Griesinger, *Mental Pathology and Therapeutics*, p. 10.

96. For the relevance of these two aspects of psychiatry's history to British alienism, see William F. Bynum, "Rationales for Therapy in British Psychiatry, 1780–1835," in Andrew Scull, ed., *Madhouses, Mad-Doctors, and Madmen: The Social History of Psychiatry in the Victorian Era* (Philadelphia: University of Pennsylvania Press, 1981), pp. 35–57.

97. George D. Sussman, "The Glut of Doctors," p. 304.

98. David H. Pinkney, *Decisive Years in France, 1840–1847* (Princeton: Princeton University Press, 1986), chap. 4.

99. L. Cerise, "Introduction," *Amp.* 1 (1843):i–xxvii.

100. Ibid., p. iii.

101. Ibid., p. viii.

102. Goldstein, *Console and Classify*, pp. 242–45.

103. Cerise, "Introduction," p. xi.

104. Claude Bernard, "Recherches anatomiques et physiologiques sur la corde du tympan pour servir à l'histoire de l'hémiplegie faciale," *Amp.* 1 (1843):408–39. See also "Quelques observations relatives à l'action de la corde du tympan. Réponse de M. Bernard à un article de M. le docteur Verga," *Amp.* 2 (1843):195–200. For Bernard on the use of hypotheses or "preconceived ideas," see his *An Introduction to the Study of Experimental Medicine*, trans. Henry Copley Green (New York: Dover, 1957), pp. 23–24.

105. Cerise, "Introduction," p. xix.

106. Ibid., p. xxvii.

107. Ibid., p. xxii.

108. Ibid., pp. xxiii–xxv.

109. L. Cerise, *Des fonctions et des maladies nerveuses dans leur rapports avec l'éducation sociale et privée moral et physique* (Paris: Baillière, 1842), pp. ix–xx.

110. L. Cerise, "Que faut-il entendre, en physiologie et en pathologie, par ces mots: Influence du moral sur le physique, influence du physique sur le moral?" *Amp.* 1 (1843):4–5.

111. Ibid., pp. 18–19.

112. L. S. Jacyna, "Medical Science and Moral Science: The Cultural Relations of Physiology in Restoration France," *History of Science* 25 (1987):111–147.

113. L. Cerise, "Que faut-il entendre," p. 18. See also P. J. B. Buchez, "Etudes sur les éléments pathogéniques de la folie," *Amp.* 6 (1854):175–96.

114. Robert Castel, *L'Ordre psychiatrique*, pp. 121–22.

115. For a critical examination of the "ego psychology" of Cousin, see P. J. B. Buchez, *Essai d'un traité complet de philosophie du point de vue du catholicisme et du progrès*, 3 vols. (Paris: Eveillard, 1838–40) 1: 147–59.

116. Ackerknecht, *Medicine at the Paris Hospital*, p. 101.

Chapter Two:
François Leuret and Medical Opposition to Moral Treatment, 1835–1850

1. For psychiatry's involvement in the publication of the *Annales d'hygiène publique et de médecine légale* and in the public hygiene movement, see Jan Ellen Goldstein, "French Psychiatry in Social and Political Context: The Formation of a New Profession, 1820–1860" (Ph.D. diss., Columbia University, 1978). See also Goldstein's *Console and Classify: The French Psychiatric Profession in the Nineteenth Century* (Cambridge: Cambridge University Press, 1987), pp. 128–47.

2. U. Trélat, "Notice sur François Leuret," *Annales d'hygiène publique et de médecine légale* 45 (1851):241–62; A. Brierre de Boismont, "Notice biographique sur M. François Leuret," *Annales médico-psychologiques* 3(1851):512–27 (hereafter cited as *Amp.*).

3. Fr. Leuret, *Fragments psychologiques sur la folie* (Paris: Crochard, 1834) (hereafter cited as Leuret, *Fragments*).

4. Brierre de Boismont, "Notice biographique sur M. François Leuret," p. 516.

5. Leuret, *Fragments*, pp. 70, 185.

6. Trélat, "Notice sur François Leuret," p. 249.

7. Leuret, *Fragments*, pp. 90–91.

8. Fr. Leuret, *Du traitement moral de la folie* (Paris: Baillière, 1840), p. 1 (hereafter cited as Leuret, *Traitement moral*).

9. Ibid., p. 66.

10. Ibid., p. 156.

11. Ibid., p. 45.

12. Ibid., pp. 49–63.

13. Ibid., p. 79.

14. Ibid., pp. 107–8.

15. A. Millet, "Nouvelles observations sur le traitement de la folie," *Archives générales de médecine* 9 (1840):249–64.

16. Leuret, *Traitement moral*, pp. 123, 129.

17. Ibid., p. 111.

18. L. Delasiauve, review of L. F. Calmeil's *Traité des maladies inflammatoires du cerveau* in *Amp.* 6 (1860):479–80.

19. For accounts of Pinel's career in psychiatry, see Dora B. Weiner, "Health and Mental Health in the Thought of Philippe Pinel: The Emergence of Psychiatry during the French Revolution," in Charles E. Rosenberg, ed., *Healing and History: Essays for George Rosen* (Kent: William Dawson, 1979), pp. 59–85; Kathleen M. Grange, "Pinel and Eighteenth-Century Psychiatry," *Bulletin of the History of Medicine* 35 (1961):442–53; Evelyn A. Woods and Eric T. Carlson, "The Psychiatry of Philippe Pinel," Ibid., pp. 14–25. See also Jan Goldstein, *Console and Classify*, pp. 64–119.

20. Philippe Pinel, *A Treatise on Insanity*, trans. D. D. Davis (Sheffield: Cadell and Davies, 1806; reprint, New York: Hafner, 1962), p. 5.

21. Goldstein, *Console and Classify*, p. 89, discussed in Andrew Scull, *Social Order/Mental Disorder: Anglo-American Psychiatry in Historical Perspective* (Berkeley: University of California Press, 1989), pp. 19–20.

22. E. Georget, *De la folie* (Paris: Crevot, 1820), pp. 245–46, 248. Cited in Robert Castel, *L'Ordre psychiatrique: L'Âge d'or de l'aliénisme* (Paris: Editions de Minuit, 1976), pp. 113–14.

23. 27 Nov. 1854 meeting of the Société médico-psychologique, *Amp.* 1 (1855):354.

24. Pierre Morel and Claude Quétel, "Les Thérapeutiques de l'aliénation mentale au 19e siècle," in Jacques Postel and Claude Quétel, eds., *Nouvelle histoire de la psychiatrie* (Toulouse: Privat, 1983), pp. 431–42; see also E. P. Poterin du Motel, "Etudes sur la melancholie et sur le traitement moral de cette maladie," *Mémoires de l'Académie royale de médecine* 21 (1857):443–527.

25. L. Lunier, "De l'emploi de la médication bromoiodurée dans le traitement de l'aliénation mentale," *Amp.* 5 (1853):89–91.

26. Leuret, *Traitement moral*, p. 68.

27. Ibid., pp. 73–74.

28. Ibid., p. 68.

29. Trélat, "Notice sur François Leuret," p. 258; Brierre de Boismont, "Notice biographique sur M. François Leuret," p. 525.

30. L. F. E. Renaudin, Review of German Medical Journals, *Amp.* 7 (1846):451–52.

31. E. Blanche, "Du danger des rigueurs corporelles dans le traitement de la folie," *Bulletin de l'Académie royale de médecine* 4 (1838–1839):79–87. Report of Pariset and Esquirol. Leuret's papers were entitled "Mémoire sur le traitement moral de la folie" and "Nouveau mémoire sur le traitement moral de la folie," *Mémoires de l'Académie royale de médecine* 7 (1838):552–76.

32. Blanche, "Du danger des rigueurs corporelles," pp. 81–83.

33. Ibid., pp. 84–85.

34. Ibid., pp. 86–87.

35. Fr. Leuret, "Mémoire sur la révulsion morale dans le traitement de la folie," *Mémoires de l'Académie royale de médecine* 9 (1841):655–71. Report of Pariset, Louis, and Double.

36. Ibid., pp. 698–89.

37. Ibid., p. 707.

38. Ibid., p. 708.

39. Ibid., p. 709.

40. Ibid., p. 710.

41. Ibid., p. 712.

42. Ibid., pp. 695–96.

43. A. Millet, "Nouvelles observations sur le traitement de la folie," pp. 252–54.

44. Ibid., pp. 250–51.

45. Michel Foucault, *Discipline and Punish: The Birth of the Prison,* trans. Alan Sheridan (New York: Vintage, 1979).

46. Leuret, *Traitement moral,* pp. 146–47.

47. *Bulletin de l'Académie royale de médecine* 6 (1840–1841):714.

48. Leuret, *Traitement moral,* p. 1.

49. George Weisz, "The Politics of Medical Professionalization in France, 1845–1848," *Journal of Social History* 12 (1978):3–30; Matthew Ramsey, "The Politics of Professional Monopoly in Nineteenth-Century Medicine: The French Model and its Rivals," in Gerald L. Geison, ed., *Professions and the French State, 1700–1900* (Philadelphia: University of Pennsylvania Press, 1984), pp. 239–40.

50. Jacques G. Petit, "Folie, langage, pouvoirs en Maine-et-Loire, 1800–1841," *Revue d'histoire moderne et contemporaine* 27 (1980): 529–64.

51. Goldstein, *Console and Classify*, pp. 200–210.

52. H. Dagonet, report for the Aubanel essay prize on the question of the dangerousness of the insane, 25 April 1870 meeting of the Société médico-psychologique, *Amp.* 4 (1870):97.

53. L. Peisse, *La Médecine et les médecins: Philosophie, doctrines, institutions, critiques, moeurs, et biographies médicales,* 2 vols. (Paris: Baillière, 1857), 2:17–18.

54. A. Lemoine, *L'Aliéné devant la philosophie, la morale, et la société* (Paris: Didier, 1862), p. 28.

55. Ibid., p. 452.

56. Ibid., p. 444.

57. Ibid., p. 453.

58. Ibid., p. 444.

59. *Amp.* 7 (1846):437–40.

60. Brierre de Boismont, "Notice biographique sur M. François Leuret," pp. 525–26.

61. Ch. Lasègue, "La Théorie du traitement moral, est-elle possible?" *Amp.* 7 (1846):388–404.

62. René Semelaigne, *Les Pionniers de la psychiatrie française avant et après Pinel,* 2 vols. (Paris: Baillière, 1930–1932), 1:302–3.

63. Ibid., 2:13–17.

64. Lemoine, *L'Aliéné,* p. 90.

65. Dr. Brochin, review of Cl. Michéa's "Influence des substances narcotiques sur le guérison de l'aliénation mentale," article published in the *Gazette médicale de Paris, Amp.* 5 (1853):687.

66. "Anatomie pathologique de cerveau des aliénés affectés de paralysie," *Amp.* 5 (1845):453–54.

67. J. André Rochoux, "Tout phénomène du domaine de la psychologie est le produit d'une action de l'encéphale et n'a pas d'autre cause," *Amp.* 8 (1846):1n. For Rochoux's offer, see *Lancette française,* 10 April 1845.

68. *Amp.* 5 (1845):454.

69. Ibid., pp. 455–57.

70. William F. Bynum, "Rationales for Therapy in British Psychiatry, 1780–1835," in Andrew Scull, ed., *Madhouses, Mad-Doctors, and Madmen: The Social History of Psychiatry in the Victorian Era* (Philadelphia: University of Pennsylvania Press, 1981), pp. 35–57.

71. For an example of the way in which Leuret's and Heinroths's views were associated, see Ferrus's comments in *Bulletin de l'Académie royale de médecine* 6 (1840–1841): 711. For Leuret's attitude toward the nineteenth-century asylum, see his *Traitement moral,* pp. 164–65 and his

"Nouveau mémoire sur le traitment moral de la folie," *Bulletin de l'Ac-adémie royale de médecine* 3 (1838–1839):204, 661; see also Claude Quétel, "Le Vote de la loi de 1838," in Postel and Quétel, *Nouvelle histoire de la psychiatrie,* p. 184.

72. Andrew T. Scull, *Museums of Madness: The Social Organization of Insanity in Nineteenth-Century England* (London: Allen Lane, 1979), p. 167; L. S. Jacyna, "Somatic Theories of Mind and the Interests of Medicine in Britain, 1850–1879," *Medical History* 26 (1982):233–58; Roger Cooter, "Phrenology and British Alienists ca. 1825–1845," in Scull, *Madhouses,* pp. 58–104.

Chapter Three:
Jacques Moreau de Tours and the Crisis of
Somaticism in French Psychiatry, 1840–1860

1. For biographical accounts of Moreau, see René Semelaigne, *Les Pionniers de la psychiatrie française avant et après Pinel,* 2 vols. (Paris: Baillière, 1930–1932), 1:294–301; also Antoine Ritti, "Eloge de Moreau (de Tours)," *Annales médico-psychologiques* 6 (1887):112–45 (hereafter cited as *Amp.*).

2. Semelaigne, *Les Pionniers,* 1:296.

3. Ritti, "Eloge de Moreau," p. 127.

4. Semelaigne, *Les Pionniers,* 1:295.

5. J. Moreau de Tours, *La Psychologie morbide dans ses rapports avec la philosophie de l'histoire ou de l'influence des névropathies sur le dynamisme intellectuel* (Paris: Masson, 1859), p. 430n (hereafter cited as Moreau, *Psychologie morbide*).

6. J. Moreau de Tours, *Hashish and Mental Illness,* ed. Helene Peters and Gabriel G. Nahas, trans. of 1845 ed. by Gordon J. Barnett (New York: Raven Press, 1973), p. 62 (hereafter cited as Moreau, *Hashish*).

7. Ibid., p. 67.

8. Ibid., p. 187.

9. Ibid., p. 193.

10. Ibid., p. 197.

11. Ibid., p. 18.

12. Ibid., p. 16.

13. Ibid., p. 135.

14. Ibid., p. 16.

15. Ibid., p. 205.

16. Ibid., pp. 16–18.

17. Ibid., p. 205.

18. Ibid., pp. 205–8.

19. Ibid., pp. 16, 196.

20. Ibid., p. 213.

21. Ibid., pp. 206–7.

22. Charles Lasègue, *Ecrits psychiatriques*, textes choisis et présentés par J. Corrage (Toulouse: Privat, 1971), p. 18.

23. Ch. Lasègue, review of Moreau's *Du haschisch et de l'aliénation mentale* in *Amp*. 7 (1846):463.

24. J. Moreau de Tours, "Mémoire sur les prodromes de la folie," read to the Paris Academy of Medicine 22 April 1851, *Amp*. 4 (1852):177.

25. Cited in Fr. Leuret, *Du traitement moral de la folie* (Paris: Baillière, 1840), p. 80 (hereafter cited as Leuret, *Traitement moral*).

26. Semelaigne, *Les Pionniers*, 1:300–301. For the similar attempt by nineteenth-century British alienists to discover new somatic remedies to bolster the conviction of medicine's value in curing insanity, see Andrew T. Scull, *Museums of Madness: The Social Organization of Insanity in Nineteenth-Century England* (London: Allen Lane, 1979), p. 170.

27. Moreau, "Mémoire sur les prodromes de la folie," p. 198.

28. Moreau, *Hashish*, p. 44.

29. Ibid., p. 19.

30. "Du délire au point de vue pathologique et anatomo-pathologique," report of Dr. Bousquet read to the Imperial Academy of Medicine 8 May 1855 and discussion thereof, *Amp*. 1 (1855):520.

31. Ibid., pp. 455–520.

32. L. Cerise, footnote to A. Royer-Collard's "Examen de la doctrine de Maine de Biran sur les rapports du physique et du moral de l'homme," *Amp*. 2 (1843):4n.

33. Fr. Leuret, *Fragments psychologiques sur la folie* (Paris: Crochard, 1834), p. 85 (hereafter cited as Leuret, *Fragments*).

34. Ibid., p. 90.

35. A. Brierre de Boismont, "Notice biographique sur M. François Leuret," *Amp*. 3 (1851):517.

36. Fr. Dubois d'Amiens, "Quelques considérations sur l'aliénation mentale au point de vue de la psychologie," meeting of the Royal Academy of Medicine, 8 April 1845, *Amp*. 6 (1845):123–31.

37. Discussion at Royal Academy of Medicine of Dubois's paper, ibid., pp. 131–33.

38. L. Cerise, Introduction to Maurice Macario's *Du sommeil, des rêves, et du somnambulisme dans l'état de santé et de maladie* (Paris: Baillière, 1857), p. xx.

39. L. F. Lélut, "Du sommeil envisagé au point de vue psychologique," *Amp*. 7 (1855):81n., 110–11.

40. Albert Lemoine, *Du sommeil au point de vue physiologique et psychologique* (Paris: Baillière, 1855), p. 3.

41. Ibid., p. vii.

42. Ibid., pp. 99–102.

43. L. Peisse, *La Médecine et les médecins: Philosophie, doctrines, institutions, critiques, moeurs, et biographies médicales*, 2 vols. (Paris: Baillière, 1857), 2:5.

44. Albert Lemoine, *L'Aliéné devant la philosophie, la morale, et la société* (Paris: Didier, 1862), p. 26.

45. Ibid., pp. 211–13.

46. "Discussion sur la folie raisonnante," 8 January 1866 meeting of the Société medico-psychologique, *Amp.* 7 (1866):383–91.

47. Moreau, *Hashish*, p. 18.

48. Ibid., pp. 106–7. His emphasis.

49. Ibid., p. 165. As Achille Foville pointed out in 1872, hallucinations were especially prominent symptoms of the mental state dubbed "monomania" or "partial delirium"; see his "Nomenclature et classification des maladies mentales," *Amp.* 8 (1872):25.

50. H. Delacroix, "Maine de Biran et l'école médico-psychologique," *Bulletin de la Société française de philosophie* 24 (1924):51–63. See also Henri F. Ellenberger, *The Discovery of the Unconscious: The History and Evolution of Dynamic Psychiatry* (New York: Basic Books, 1970), p. 403. For Maine de Biran's place in nineteenth-century French philosophy, see Emile Brehier, *The Nineteenth Century: The Period of Systems 1800–1850*, trans. Wade Baskin (Chicago: University of Chicago Press, 1968), pp.42–62.

51. L. F. A. Maury, *Le Sommeil et les rêves* (Paris: Didier, 1862), p. 97.

52. Lemoine, *L'Aliéné*, pp. 130–31.

53. J. Moreau de Tours, "De l'identité de l'état de rêve et de la folie," *Amp.* 1 (1855):387–88.

54. J. André Rochoux, "Tout phénomène du domain de la psychologie est le produit d'une action de l'encéphale et n'a pas d'autre cause," *Amp.* 8 (1846): p. 2n.

55. Lemoine, *L'Aliéné*, p. 25.

56. L. F. A. Maury, *Souvenirs d'un homme de lettres*. Bibliothèque de l'Institut de France, MS. 2656, vol. 19, DCCXIX, p. 1.

57. For Cousin's influence on French philosophy in the last century, see Thomas Michael Telzrow, "The 'Watchdogs': French Academic Philosophy in the Nineteenth Century: The Case of Paul Janet" (Ph.D. diss., University of Wisconsin, 1973).

58. Royer-Collard, "Examen."

59. Telzrow, "The 'Watchdogs'," p. 43.

60. J. Moreau de Tours, "De la folie au point de vue pathologique et anatomo-pathologique," *Amp.* 7 (1855):11–40.

61. J. Moreau de Tours, "De l'identité de l'état de rêve et de la folie," *Amp.* 1 (1855):361–408.

62. Moreau, "De la folie" pp. 12–13.

63. For another example of this ploy, see Jules Falret, "Discussion sur la folie raisonnante," 8 January 1866 meeting of the Société médico-psychologique, *Amp.* 7 (1866):386. The reasons why many alienists—though not all—liked to associate insanity with delirium were clear to most physicians of the time. The French term *"délire"* is not the same as the English term "delirium." *Délire* for most nineteenth-century French physicians referred to a change of the psyche involving all the mental faculties at an elementary level, a process more fundamental than simply a delusional idea and closely associated with the passivity of involuntarism. Since one of the best examples of *délire* was the psychological disarray of dreaming, defining insanity as virtually synonymous with *délire* served many of the same purposes as equating insanity and dreaming: it reinforced the notion that the psychological phenomena of mental illness derived from a profound physiological disorder of the brain, and hence were genuinely pathological and recognizable only to physicians. For an explanation of the French psychiatric use of the term *délire*, see G. E. Berrios, "Obsessional Disorders during the Nineteenth Century: Terminological and Classificatory Issues," in W. F. Bynum, Roy Porter, and Michael Shepherd, eds., *The Anatomy of Madness: Essays in the History of Psychiatry*, 2 vols. (London and New York: Tavistock, 1985), 1:184n82. See also Jan Goldstein, *Console and Classify: The French Psychiatric Profession in the Nineteenth Century* (Cambridge: Cambridge University Press, 1987), pp. 176–77, 195, 263.

64. Moreau, "De la folie" p. 17.

65. J. B. E. Bousquet, "Du délire au point de vue pathologique et anatomo-pathologique," *Amp.* 1 (1855):448–55.

66. Peisse, *La Médecine*, 2:7–8.

67. Leuret, *Traitement moral*, pp. 66, 110–11.

68. "Discussion sur le rapport de M. Bousquet," *Amp.* 1 (1855):497.

69. Ibid., pp. 455–70.

70. Delacroix, "Maine de Biran."

71. *Amp.* 1 (1855):507.

72. Ibid., p. 487.

73. Ibid., p. 503.

74. Ibid., p. 497.

75. Ibid., p. 501.

76. Ibid., p. 506.

77. See E. Carrière's review of J. Moreau de Tours, "Un chapître oublié de la pathologie mentale," *Amp*. 2 (1850):441.

78. Moreau, *Psychologie morbide*, p. 106.

79. Moreau, "Mémoire sur les prodromes de la folie," pp. 175–98.

80. J. Moreau de Tours, "De la prédisposition héréditaire aux affections cérébrales. Existe-t-il des signes particuliers auxquels on puisse reconnaître cette prédisposition?" *Amp*. 4 (1852):119–20, 449.

81. Moreau, "Mémoire sur les prodromes de la folie," *Amp*. 3 (1851):503.

82. Moreau, *Psychologie morbide*, p. 255.

83. Ibid., pp. 101–102.

84. Ibid., p. 138.

85. Ibid., p. 490.

86. Ibid., p. 106.

87. For recognition of this insight of Moreau's, see H. Bonnet, *L'Aliéné devant lui-même, l'appréciation légale, la législation, les systêmes, la société, et la famille* (Paris: Masson, 1865), p. 131.

88. Moreau, *Psychologie morbide*, p. 308.

89. Moreau, "De la prédisposition," pp. 452–53.

90. *Amp*. 1 (1855):458, 478–79, 503.

91. "Anatomie pathologique du cerveau des aliénés affectés de paralysie," *Amp*. 5 (1845):455.

92. Pierre Morel and Claude Quétel, "Les Thérapeutiques de l'aliénation mentale au 19e siècle," in Jacques Postel and Claude Quétel, eds., *Nouvelle histoire de la psychiatrie* (Toulouse: Privat, 1983), pp. 431–32.

93. *Amp*. 1 (1855):479. See also P. A. Piorry, *De l'hérédité dans les maladies* (Paris: Bury, 1840).

94. L. S. Jacyna, "Somatic Theories of Mind and the Interests of Medicine in Britain, 1850–1879," *Medical History* 26 (1982):244.

95. Moreau, *Hashish*, p. 206n.

96. David Ingleby, "Mental Health and Social Order," in Stanley Cohen and Andrew Scull, eds., *Social Control and the State: Historical and Comparative Essays* (Oxford: Martin Robertson; New York: St. Martin's Press, 1983), p. 165.

97. Eliot Freidson, *Profession of Medicine: A Study of the Sociology of Applied Knowledge* (New York: Dodd, Mead, 1970); Scull, *Museums of Madness*.

98. M. Legrand, review of Moreau's *Psychologie morbide* in *Union médicale*, 20 September 1859, pp. 539–40.

99. 26 November 1860 meeting of the Société médico-psychologique, *Amp*. 7 (1861):176.

Chapter Four:
Alienism and the Psychiatric Search
for a Professional Identity: The Société
médico-psychologique, 1840–1870

1. J. Baillarger, "Association des médicins des hospices d'aliénés en Angleterre. De l'utilité que pourrait avoir une association semblable parmi les médecins français," *Annales médico-psychologiques* 1 (1843): 181–83 (hereafter cited as *Amp.*).

2. René Charpentier, "La Naissance de la Société médico-psychologique," *Amp.* 2 (1952):43.

3. *Amp.* 6 (1845):196–222.

4. *Amp.* 7 (1846):467–72. For the importance of statistics for U.S. asylum superintendents in their efforts to organize an association of psychiatrists, see Constance M. McGovern, *Masters of Madness: Social Origins of the American Psychiatric Profession* (Hanover, N.H.: University Press of New England, 1985), pp. 69–74.

5. See Théophile Archambault, review of J.-B. Cazauvieilh's *Du suicide, de l'aliénation mentale et des crimes contre les personnes* in *Amp.* 1 (1843):171. See also Louis Chevalier, *Labouring Classes and Dangerous Classes in Paris during the First Half of the Nineteenth Century*, trans. Frank Jellinek (New York: Howard Fertig, 1973), pp. 41–53; Erwin H. Ackerknecht, *Medicine at the Paris Hospital, 1794–1848* (Baltimore: Johns Hopkins Press, 1967), pp. 152–53.

6. Jan Ellen Goldstein, "French Psychiatry in Social and Political Context: The Formation of a New Profession, 1820–1860" (Ph.D. diss., Columbia University, 1978), pp. 371–74.

7. *Amp.* 7 (1846):472n.

8. David H. Pinkney, *Decisive Years in France, 1840–1847* (Princeton: Princeton University Press, 1986), chap. 4.

9. See George D. Sussman, "The Glut of Doctors in Mid-Nineteenth-Century France," *Comparative Studies in Social History* 19 (1977): 287–304; also George Weisz, "The Politics of Medical Professionalization in France, 1845–1848," *Journal of Social History* 12 (1978): 3–30.

10. C. E. Bourdin, *Etudes médico-psychologiques: Cerise, sa vie et ses oeuvres* (Paris: G. Jousset, 1972), p. 11. For the importance of the idea of association in post-1815 French society, see K. Steven Vincent, *Pierre-Joseph Proudhon and the Rise of French Republican Socialism* (New York and Oxford: Oxford University Press, 1984), pp. 127–45.

11. Charpentier, "La Naissance," p. 44.

12. J. Baillarger, "Fondation de la Société médico-psychologique," *Amp.* 11 (1848):1–2.

13. "Société médico-psychologique: Règlement," ibid., pp. 3–8.

14. Jan Goldstein, *Console and Classify: The French Psychiatric Profession in the Nineteenth Century* (Cambridge: Cambridge University Press, 1987), pp. 340–41.

15. Charpentier, "La Naissance," p. 45.

16. "Nouveau règlement de la Société médico-psychologique" and "Rapport sur les modifications à introduire dans le project de règlement de la Société médico-psychologique," *Amp.* 4 (1852):226–34.

17. Th. Ribot, "Philosophy in France," *Mind* 2 (1877):368.

18. 30 Nov. 1863 meeting of the Société médico-psychologique, *Amp.* 3 (1864):134.

19. Cited in George Boas, *French Philosophies of the Romantic Period* (New York: Russell and Russell, 1964), pp. 215–16.

20. Ibid., p. 201.

21. Cited in Emile Brehier, *The History of Philosophy: The Nineteenth Century: Period of Systems 1800–1850*, trans. Wade Baskin (Chicago: University of Chicago Press, 1968), p. 91.

22. Philip A. Bertocci, *Jules Simon: Republican Anticlericalism and Cultural Politics in France 1848–1886* (Columbia: University of Missouri Press, 1978), p. 117.

23. *Amp.* 10 (1867):493.

24. L. S. Jacyna, "Medical Science and Moral Science: The Cultural Relations of Physiology in Restoration France," *History of Science* 25 (1987):111–46.

25. Ian R. Dowbiggin, "The Professional, Sociopolitical, and Cultural Dimensions of Psychiatric Theory in France 1840–1900" (Ph.D. diss., University of Rochester, 1986), chap. 3.

26. E. Saisset, "Renaissance du voltairianisme," *Revue des deux mondes* 9 (1845):377–408.

27. L. F. A. Maury, *Souvenirs d'un homme de lettres*. Bibliothèque de l'Institut de France, MS. 2650, vol. 4, p. 21. Hereafter cited as Maury, *Souvenirs*.

28. L. Cerise, "Quelques mots sur la liberté de discussion dans les *Annales médico-psychologiques*," *Amp.* 7 (1846):157.

29. For example, see L. F. Lélut, "De l'amulette de Pascal: Etude sur les rapports de la santé de ce grand homme à son génie," *Amp.* 5 (1845):1–15, 157–80; "Formule des rapports du cerveau à la pensée," *Amp.* 1 (1843):185–207; "Cadre de la philosophie de l'homme," *Amp.* 3 (1844):157–64. Also see L. F. A. Maury, "L'Amulette de Pascal, pour servir à l'histoire des hallucinations," *Amp.* 8 (1846):285–99; review of L. F. Calmeil's *De la folie considérée sous le point de vue pathologique, philosophique, historique, et judiciare depuis la renaissance des sciences en Europe jusqu'au dix-neuvième siècle* in *Amp.* 7 (1846):110–33; re-

view of A. Brierre de Boismont's *Des hallucinations, ou histoire raisonnée des apparitions, des visions, des songes, de l'extase, des rêves, du magnétisme et du somnambulisme*, in *Amp*. 5 (1845):300–311.

30. A. Brierre de Boismont, *Hallucinations: Or, the Rational History of Apparitions, Visions, Dreams, Ecstasy, Magnetism and Somnambulism*, 1st American ed. from 2nd enlarged French ed. of 1851 (Philadelphia: Lindsay and Blackiston, 1853), p. 361.

31. L. Delasiauve, "Société médico-psychologique: Ses phases, ses travaux," *Gazette hébdomadaire de médecine et de chirurgie*, 7 August 1857.

32. Georges Collet, "Les Fondateurs de la Société médico-psychologique," *Amp*. 2 (1952):53.

33. René Semelaigne, *Les Pionniers de la psychiatrie française avant et après Pinel*, 2 vols. (Paris: Baillière, 1930–1932), 1:344.

34. A. Ritti, "Cinquantenaire de la Société médico-psychologique," *Amp*. 16 (1902):37.

35. Maury, *Souvenirs*, MS. 2650, vol. 4, pp. 20–21, 350.

36. Ibid.; see also MS. 2647, vol. 1, pp. 1–2.

37. Barbara Patricia Petri, *The Historical Thought of P. J. B. Buchez* (Washington: Catholic University of America Press, 1958), p. 15.

38. P. J. B. Buchez, *Essai d'un traité complet de philosophie du point de vue du catholicisme et du progrès*, 3 vols. (Paris: Eveillard, 1838–1840), 2:418.

39. Maury, *Souvenirs*, MS. 2650, vol. 4, p. 20.

40. P. J. B. Buchez, "Quelques mots de philosophie à propos d'aliénation mentale," *Amp*. 4 (1852):509–19.

41. Léon Rostan, *Exposition des principes de l'organicisme précédée de réflexions sur l'incredulité en matière de médecine*, 3rd ed. (Paris: Asselin, 1864), pp. 160–70.

42. L. F. E. Renaudin, *Etudes médico-psychologiques sur l'aliénation mentale* (Paris: Baillière, 1854), pp. 2–3.

43. A. Lemoine, *L'Aliéné devant la philosophie, la morale, et la société* (Paris: Didier, 1862), pp. 26–27.

44. L. Peisse, *La Médecine et les médecins: Philosophie, doctrines, institutions, critiques, moeurs, et biographies médicales*, 2 vols. (Paris: Baillière, 1857), 2:5.

45. 27 Dec. 1869 meeting of the Société médico-psychologique, *Amp*. 3 (1870):305.

46. 27 Jan. 1868 meeting of the Société médico-psychologique, *Amp*. 11 (1868):280.

47. For the relationship between Girard de Cailleux and Hausmann, see Gerard Bleandonu and Guy Le Gaufey, "The Creation of the Insane Asylums of Auxerre and Paris," in Robert Forster and Orest Ranum, eds.,

Deviants and the Abandoned in French Society, trans. Elborg Forster and Patricia M. Ranum, 4 vols. (Baltimore and London: Johns Hopkins University Press, 1978), 4:180–212; for Hausmann's role in the rebuilding of Paris during the Second Empire, see David H. Pinkney, *Napoleon III and the Rebuilding of Paris* (Princeton: Princeton University Press, 1958); for the political strategy behind the reconstruction of Paris, see Ibid., pp. 35–39.

48. Jan Goldstein, " 'Moral Contagion': A Professional Ideology of Medecine and Psychiatry in Eighteenth- and Nineteenth-Century France," in Gerald L. Geison, ed., *Professions and the French State, 1700–1900* (Philadelphia: University of Pennsylvania Press, 1984), pp. 181–222.

49. Maury, *Souvenirs*, MS. 2648, vol. 2, p. 349.

Chapter Five:
French Alienism and Antipsychiatry,
1860–1900

1. Robert Castel, *L 'Ordre psychiatrique: L 'Âge d'or de l'aliénisme* (Paris: Editions de Minuit, 1976), p. 268.

2. Maurice Desruelles, "Histoire des projets de révision de la loi du 30 Juin 1838," *Annales médico-psychologiques* 1 (1938):592 (hereafter cited as *Amp.*).

3. *Amp.* 5 (1865):137.

4. I use the term "antipsychiatry" to describe the skepticism toward the social and medical usefulness of asylum medicine shared by spokespersons of the liberal left and the clerical/monarchical right, an attitude that peaked in the 1860s. I employ the term deliberately to draw attention to the similarities between it and the "antipsychiatry" of the 1960s associated with Thomas Szasz, R. D. Laing, Erving Goffman, Michel Foucault, and others. While nineteenth-century French antipsychiatry may not have developed alternative models of mental illness as systematically as did the antipsychiatrists of the 1960s, the fact that there were clerical interests behind much of the attack on asylum psychiatry in the 1860s suggests that at an elementary level both movements shared a "psychodynamic" approach to insanity that stressed the psychological mechanisms underlying madness and de-emphasized its physical nature.

5. Dr. Caffe, "De l'interdiction des aliénés," Ibid. 3 (1864):201.

6. Ibid., p. 203.

7. H. Bonnet, "Les Aliénés devant la société," *Amp.* 3 (1864):160.

8. 28 Dec. 1863 meeting of the Société médico-psychologique, *Amp.* 3 (1864):280–81.

9. A. Brierre de Boismont, "Appréciation médico-légale du régime actuel des aliénés en France à l'occasion de la loi de 1838," *Amp*. 6 (1865):59.

10. Ibid., p. 86.

11. Jan Goldstein, *Console and Classify: The French Psychiatric Profession in the Nineteenth Century* (Cambridge: Cambridge University Press, 1987), p. 281.

12. Ibid., pp. 353–54.

13. H. Dagonet, "Loi de Juin 1838: Asiles d'aliénés," *Amp*. 5 (1865): 216–20.

14. Th. Rousselin, "De l'utilité de la séquestration au début des maladies mentales au point de vue du double intêret de la société et de l'aliéné," Ibid., pp. 455–70.

15. C. Pinel, "Quelques mots sur les asiles d'aliénés et la loi de 1838 à propos d'une pétition au sénat," *Journal de médecine mentale* 4 (1864): 144–58.

16. Théophile Roussel, *Notes et documents concernant la législation française et les législations étrangères sur les aliénés. Annexe au procès-verbal de la séance du 20 mai 1884. Commission relative à la révision de la loi du 30 juin 1838 sur les aliénés*, 2 vols. (Paris: P. Mouillot, 1884), 1:205n (hereafter cited as Roussel, *Notes*).

17. Th. Rousselin and L. Lunier, "Etude médico-légale sur l'état mental de M. du Puyparlier," *Amp*. 4 (1870):56–89.

18. Drs. Baume and Lafitte, "Les Aliénés et la presse," Ibid. 3 (1870): 57–79.

19. Peter McCandless, "Liberty and Lunacy: The Victorians and Wrongful Confinement," in Andrew T. Scull, ed., *Madhouses, Mad-Doctors, and Madmen: The Social History of Psychiatry in the Victorian Era* (Philadelphia: University of Pennsylvania Press, 1981), p. 357.

20. See Robert A. Nye, *Crime, Madness, and Politics in Modern France: The Medical Concept of National Decline* (Princeton: Princeton University Press, 1984).

21. Baume and Lafitte, "Les Aliénés et la presse," p. 77.

22. Ibid., p. 75.

23. Ibid., p. 73.

24. Roussel, *Notes*, pp. 298–99.

25. Goldstein, *Console and Classify*, pp. 352–53.

26. Rousselin and Lunier, "Etude médico-légale," pp. 81–89.

27. "Nécrologie," *Amp*. 5 (1887):168–69.

28. For an account of Gheel, see William L. Parry-Jones, "The Model of the Gheel Colony and its Influence on the Nineteenth-Century Asylum System in Britain," in Scull, *Madhouses*, pp. 201–17.

29. For a lengthy description of and answer to the allegations of Turck's petition, see J. B. Parchappe, 27 Nov. 1865 meeting of the Société médico-psychologique, *Amp*. 7 (1866):105–50.

30. Castel, *L'Ordre*, p. 270.

31. Rousselin and Lunier, "Etude médico-légale," pp. 72–73.

32. H. Bonnet, "La Vérité sur l'affaire Jeanson," *Amp*. 3 (1870): 230–62.

33. B. A. Morel, "La Vérité sur l'affaire Jeanson: Réponse à M. le Dr. Bonnet," Ibid., pp. 420–46.

34. Charles E. Rosenberg, *The Trial of the Assassin Guiteau: Psychiatry and Law in the Gilded Age* (Chicago and London: The University of Chicago Press, 1968).

35. Bonnet, "La Vérité," pp. 237, 259.

36. H. Thulié, "Lettre à M. le Dr. Motet," Ibid., pp. 522–25.

37. See "Pétitions relatives à la législation des aliénés," *Amp*. 12 (1868):162–67.

38. "Commission chargée d'étudier les questions relatives à le loi de 1838," *Amp*. 1 (1869):363–66.

39. "Loi sur les aliénés," *Amp*. 4 (1870):346–48.

40. Desruelles, "Histoire des projets," pp. 596–97.

41. "Loi sur les aliénés," p. 347.

42. Castel, *L'Ordre*, p. 268.

43. Roussel, *Notes*.

44. Goldstein, *Console and Classify*, p. 365.

45. A. Giraud, "Chronique: La Proposition de loi sur le régime des aliénés présentée par M. Reinach, député," *Amp*. 13 (1891):177–92.

46. Nye, *Crime*, pp. 236–47.

47. Ibid. p. 241.

48. Desruelles, "Histoire des projets," pp. 600–601.

49. René Semelaigne, *Les Pionniers de la psychiatrie française avant et après Pinel*, 2 vols. (Paris: Baillière, 1930–1932), 1:235; 2:212–13. See also the 25 May 1874 meeting of the Société médico-psychologique, *Amp*. 12 (1874):270–72.

50. H. Bonnet, "La Baronne (à l'Odéon). Lettre à M. L'Inspecteur général, Lunier," *Amp*. 8 (1872):73–83.

51. Roussel, *Notes*, 1:212; see also L. Lunier's review of Ambroise Tardieu's *Etude médico-légale sur la folie* in *Amp*. 9 (1873):531.

52. *Amp*. 5 (1865):124.

53. *Amp*. 6 (1865):451.

54. *Amp*. 5 (1865):249.

55. Ibid., p. 288.

56. Ibid., p. 109.

57. *Amp*. 1 (1869):85–113. See also Ian R. Dowbiggin, "French Pychi-

atric Attitudes Towards the Dangers Posed by the Insane ca. 1870," in Andrew T. Scull and Steven Spitzer, eds., *Research in Law, Deviance and Social Control* 9 (1988):87–111.

58. H. Belloc, 26 Apr. 1869 meeting of the Société médico-psychologique, *Amp*. 2 (1869):84.

59. L. Lunier, "Des aliénés dangereux; étudiés au triple point de vue clinique, administratif, et médico-légale," *Amp*. 2 (1869):169–96.

60. Ibid., p. 171.

61. *Amp*. 1 (1869):294–97.

62. For example, see the remarks of A. Motet, 14 Nov. 1864 meeting of the Société médico-psychologique, *Amp*. 5 (1865):115.

63. A. Foville, 16 Jan. 1865 meeting of the Société, *Amp*. 5 (1865): 342; H. Dagonet, report on the Prix Aubanel, 25 Apr. 1870, *Amp*. 4 (1870):97.

64. 30 Oct. 1865 meeting of the Société, *Amp*. 6 (1865):453.

65. *Amp*. 1 (1869):88.

66. *Amp*. 2 (1869):87.

67. *Amp*. 8 (1872):73–83.

68. *Amp*. 6 (1887):333–34.

Chapter Six:
Hereditarianism, the Clinic, and Psychiatric Practice in Nineteenth-Century France

1. See J. E. D. Esquirol, *Mental Maladies: A Treatise on Insanity*, trans. E. K. Hunt (Philadelphia: Lea and Blanchard, 1845), p. 47; and J. Baillarger, "Recherches statistiques sur l'hérédité de la folie," *Annales médico-psychologiques* 3 (1844):328–39 (hereafter cited as *Amp*.).

2. Prosper Lucas, *Traité philosophique et physiologique de l'hérédité naturelle dans les états de santé et de maladie du système nerveux*, 2 vols. (Paris: Baillière, 1847–1850) (hereafter cited as Lucas, *Traité*).

3. Ibid., 1: vii, xx, 179–90.

4. For example, see Th. Ribot, *Heredity: A Psychological Study of its Phenomena, Laws, Causes, and Consequences* (New York: Appleton, 1875), p. 213 (hereafter cited as Ribot, *Heredity*).

5. U. Trélat, "Des causes de la folie," *Amp*. 2 (1856):7–23, 174–90.

6. L. F. E. Renaudin, "Observations sur les recherches statistiques relatives à l'aliénation mentale," *Amp*. 2 (1856):356–57, 496–97.

7. Françoise M. C. Constant, "Introduction à la vie et à l'oeuvre de B.-A. Morel (1809–73)" (Medical Thesis, Cochin-Port Royal, 1970); see also Ruth Friedlander, "B. A. Morel and the Theory of Degenerescence: The Introduction of Anthropology into Psychiatry" (Ph.D. diss., University of California at San Francisco, 1973).

8. B. A. Morel, *Traité des dégénérescences physiques, intellectuelles, et morales de l'espèce humaine* (Paris: Baillière, 1857), p. 565 (hereafter cited as Morel, *Traité*).

9. Ibid., pp. 322–23.

10. P. J. B. Buchez, "Rapport fait à la Société médico-psychologique sur le *Traité des dégénérescences physiques, intellectuelles et morales de l'espèce humaine et des causes qui les produisent*," *Amp*. 3 (1857):457.

11. *Amp*. 7 (1861):176.

12. G. Doutrebente, "Etude généalogique sur les aliénés héréditaires," *Amp*. 2 (1869):197–237, 369–94.

13. *Amp*. 10 (1868):273–74.

14. *Amp*. 11 (1868):116–17.

15. *Union médicale* 28 (1851):113–15.

16. A. Brierre de Boismont, "Morel: Fragments de son oeuvre en aliénation mentale, l'hérédité morbide, les dégénérescences," Ibid. 84 (1874):25–35; idem, "Exposé des travaux du docteur Morel sur la médecine légale des aliénés," *Annales d'hygiène publique et de médecine légale* 41 (1874):184–97 (hereafter cited as *Ann. d'hygiène*).

17. A. Brierre de Boismont, "L'Hérédité au point de vue de la médecine légale et de l'hygiène," *Ann. d'hygiène* 43 (1875):169–95.

18. P. Serieux, *Valentin Magnan: Sa vie et son oeuvre 1835–1916* (Paris: Masson, 1918), p. 2.

19. Ibid., p. 58.

20. Ibid., p. 66.

21. 31 May 1886 meeting of Société médico-psychologique, *Amp*. 4 (1886):255, 258.

22. For the debates of the Société on the physical, intellectual, and moral signs of hereditary insanity, see *Amp*. 2 (1885), 3 (1886), and 4 (1886).

23. Ch. Féré, "La Famille névropathique," *Archives de neurologie* 7 (1884):1–43, 173–91.

24. Dr. Charpentier, "Du rôle de la profession dans le développement de l'aliénation mentale," *Amp*. 11 (1883):314–25.

25. J. Dejerine, *L'Hérédité dans les maladies du système nerveux* (Paris: Asselin et Houzeau, 1886), pp. xiv–xv.

26. Ch. Féré, "La Famille névropathique," p. 7.

27. Doutrebente, "Etude généalogique sur les aliénés héréditaires," p. 211.

28. *Amp*. 4 (1886):97.

29. Ibid., p. 101.

30. 29 March 1886 meeting of the Société médico-psychologique, Ibid., p. 95.

31. Ibid., p. 255.

32. 27 July 1885 meeting of the Société, *Amp.* 3 (1886), p. 97.

33. 31 Jan. 1887 meeting of the Société, *Amp.* 6 (1887):438.

34. A. Planés, "Mouvement de l'aliénation mentale à Paris (1872–1885)," *Amp.* 5 (1887):235.

35. 25 October 1886 meeting of the Société, ibid., p. 123. Daniel Pick, in his *Faces of Degeneration: A European Disorder, c. 1848–c.1918* (Cambridge: Cambridge University Press, 1989), argues eloquently that degeneracy was an idea that resisted strict definitions and "was never successfully reduced to a fixed axiom or theory" (ibid., p. 7). Its implications were often contradictory, mainly because "nobody was able to agree precisely on what it meant" (ibid., p. 8). While Pick is ultimately more interested in the wider cultural, political, and social uses of the language of degeneration, most of what he says applies to its medical use.

36. Yvette Conry, *L'Introduction du Darwinisme en France au XIXe siècle* (Paris: Librairie philosophique J. Vrin, 1974), p. 328. Cited in Robert A. Nye, *Crime, Madness, and Politics in Modern France: The Medical Concept of National Decline* (Princeton: Princeton University Press, 1984), p. 129 (hereafter cited as Nye, *Crime*).

37. Ola Andersson, *Studies in the Prehistory of Psychoanalysis* (Stockholm, Sweden: Bokförlaget, 1962), p. 37n. As Pick has argued, degeneration "explained everything and nothing"; at the level of discourse, it was so eclectic that it could unite people from vastly different political, social, and medical positions. See Pick, *Faces of Degeneration*, p. 8.

38. B. A. Morel, "Discussion sur la classification de la folie," *Amp.* 7 (1861):176.

39. L. Lunier, review of U. Trélat's *La Folie lucide étudiée et considérée au point de vue de la famille et de la société*, in *Amp.* 7 (1861):548–664.

40. H. Dagonet, "L'Aliénation mentale chez les dégénérés psychiques," *Amp.* 14 (1891):355–56.

41. *Amp.* 15 (1876):433–53.

42. 28 June 1886 meeting of the Société médico-psychologique, *Amp.* 4 (1886):271.

43. Ibid., p. 280.

44. Ch. Lasègue, "Morel—Sa vie médicale et ses oeuvres," *Archives générales de médecine* 21 (1873):589–600.

45. J. Falret, "Des anomalies physiques associées aux désordres de l'intelligence," *Amp.* 15 (1876):413–14.

46. *Amp.* 6 (1887):439.

47. Eliot Freidson, *Profession of Medicine: A Study of the Sociology of Applied Knowledge* (New York: Dodd, Mead, and Co., 1970), p. 248.

48. P. J. B. Buchez, "Discussion sur la classification de la folie," *Amp.* 7 (1861):328–30.

49. B. A. Morel, *Traité des maladies mentales* (Paris: Masson, 1860), p. ix (hereafter cited as Morel, *Maladies*).

50. 13 Dec. 1869 meeting of the Société médico-psychologique, *Amp.* 3 (1870):282.

51. H. Legrand du Saulle, "Les Signes physiques des folies raisonnantes," *Amp.* 15 (1876):433.

52. Prosper Despine, *Etude sur les facultés intellectuelles et morales dans leur état normal et dans manifestations anomales chez les aliénés et chez les criminels*, 3 vols. (Paris: F. Savy, 1868), 2:37.

53. Ribot, *Heredity*, pp. 264–67.

54. Despine, *Etude sur les facultés*, 1:398–99.

55. Brierre de Boismont, "L'Hérédité au point de vue de la médecine légale et de l'hygiène," p. 193.

56. Ibid., p. 194.

57. Roger Smith, "The Background of Physiological Psychology in Natural Philosophy," *History of Science* 11 (1973):75–123, especially pp. 86–87.

58. E. Marcé, *Traité pratique des maladies mentales* (Paris: Baillière, 1862), p. 34. See also Robert Castel, *L'Ordre psychiatrique: L'Âge d'or de l'aliénisme* (Paris: Editions de Minuit, 1976), p. 277n (hereafter cited as Castel, *L'Ordre*). For similar attitudes in British psychiatry in the last century, see Michael J. Clark, "The Rejection of Psychological Approaches to Mental Disorder in late Nineteenth-Century British Psychiatry," in Andrew Scull, ed., *Madhouses, Mad-Doctors, and Madmen: The Social History of Psychiatry in the Victorian Era* (Philadelphia: University of Pennsylvania Press, 1981), pp. 271–312 (hereafter cited as Scull, *Madhouses*).

59. Jules Falret, Introduction to his translation of W. Griesinger's "La Pathologie mentale au point de vue de l'école somatique allemande," *Amp.* 5 (1865):4; see also William F. Bynum, "Rationales for Therapy in British Psychiatry, 1780–1825," in Scull, *Madhouses*, p. 52.

60. 27 July 1885 meeting of the Société médico-psychologique, *Amp.* 3 (1886):91–99.

61. Smith, "The Background of Physiological Psychology," p. 87.

62. For example, see J. Luys, *Traité clinique et pratique des maladies mentales* (Paris: A. Delahaye and E. Lecrosnier, 1881), p. 229; H. Dagonet, *Traité des maladies mentales*, 3rd ed. (Paris: Baillière, 1894), p. 130.

63. Claude Quétel, "La Vie quotidienne d'un asile d'aliénés à la fin du XIXe siècle," in Jacques Postel and Claude Quétel, eds., *Nouvelle histoire de la psychiatrie* (Toulouse: Privat, 1983), pp. 443–49 (hereafter cited as Postel and Quétel, *Nouvelle histoire*).

64. Clark, "Rejection of Psychological Approaches," pp. 292–301.

65. J. P. Falret, "De l'enseignement clinique des maladies mentales," *Amp.* 1 (1849):576–77.

66. L. Lunier, "De l'isolement des aliénés considéré comme moyen de traitement et comme mesure d'ordre public," *Amp.* 5 (1871):32.

67. H. Bonnet, *L'Aliéné devant lui-même, l'appréciation légale, la législation, les systèmes, la société, et la famille* (Paris: Masson, 1865), p. 17.

68. Robert Castel, "Moral Treatment: Mental Therapy and Social Control in the Nineteenth Century," trans. Peter Miller, in Stanley Cohen and Andrew Scull, eds., *Social Control and the State: Historical and Comparative Essays* (Oxford: Martin Robertson; New York: St. Martin's Press, 1983), 248–66.

69. L. Lunier, "Des placements volontaires dans les asiles d'aliénés: Etude sur les législations française et étrangères," *Amp.* 12 (1868):84.

70. H. Girard de Cailleux, "Considérations générales sur l'ensemble du service des aliénés du département de la Seine," *Amp.* 7 (1861):276.

71. Nancy Tomes, *A Generous Confidence: Thomas Story Kirkbride and the Art of Asylum–Keeping, 1840–1883* (Cambridge: Cambridge University Press, 1984), pp. 221–23. For the clerical technique of consolation and the consoling function of French psychiatry in the nineteenth century, see Jan Goldstein, *Console and Classify: The French Psychiatric Profession in the Nineteenth Century* (Cambridge: Cambridge University Press, 1987), especially pp. 202–8.

72. Freidson, *Profession of Medicine*, pp. 252–55. See also Andrew T. Scull, *Museums of Madness: The Social Organization of Insanity in Nineteenth-Century England* (London: Allen Lane, 1979), chap. 4.

73. 14 Nov. 1864 meeting of the Société médico-psychologique, *Amp.* 5 (1865):119.

74. 16 Jan. 1865 meeting of the Société, ibid., p. 354.

75. H. Bonnet, "Les Aliénés devant la société," *Amp.* 3 (1864): 163–64n.

76. Théophile Roussel, *Notes et documents concernant la législation française et les législations étrangères sur les aliénés. Annexe au procès-verbal de la séance du 20 mai 1884. Commission relative à la révision de la loi du 30 juin 1838 sur les aliénés.* 2 vols. (Paris: P. Mouillot, 1884), 1:239.

77. L. Lunier, "De l'isolement des aliénés," p. 32.

78. Albert Lemoine, *L' Aliéné devant la philosophie, la morale, et la société* (Paris: Didier, 1862), pp. 470–71. See also Despine, *Etude sur les facultés*, pp. 109–11.

79. Bonnet, *L'Aliéné*, p. 17.

80. L. F. E. Renaudin, *Etudes médico-psychologiques sur l'aliénation mentale* (Paris: Baillière, 1854), pp. 2–3, 10.

81. See Kathleen M. Grange, "Pinel and Eighteenth-Century Psychiatry," *Bulletin of the History of Medicine* 35 (1961):449.

82. B. A. Morel, 1 March 1846 letter to Dr. Ferrus, *Amp.* 7 (1846): 368.

83. Morel, *Traité*, p. 567.

84. Andrew T. Scull, "The Social History of Psychiatry in the Victorian Era," in Scull, *Madhouses*, p. 8.

85. Morel, *Traité*, p. 77.

86. Ibid.; see also Castel, *L'Ordre*, pp. 279–83.

87. Morel, *Traité*, pp. 685–87.

88. P. Berthier, "Des causes de l'encombrement des asiles d'aliénés et des remèdes à y apporter," *Amp.* 7 (1866):368–78.

89. A. Brierre de Boismont, "Morel: Fragments de son oeuvre en aliénation mentale, l'hérédité morbide, les dégénérescences," *Union médicale* 84 (1874):34.

90. Morel, *Traité*, p. 461.

91. Ibid., p. xii.

92. Ibid., pp. 77–78.

93. Ibid., p. 685.

94. Castel, *L'Ordre*, p. 283.

95. Morel, *Traité*, chap. 1.

96. Ibid., p. 589.

97. Ibid., p. 523.

98. 25 May 1868 meeting of the Société médico-psychologique, *Amp.* 11 (1868):289–90.

99. Ibid., p. 290.

100. Doutrebente, "Etude généalogique sur les aliénés héréditaires," pp. 197–237, 369–94.

101. A. Motet, report on Doutrebente's "Etude généalogique sur les aliénés héréditaires," *Amp.* 2 (1869):148–54. See also U. Trélat, *La folie lucide, étudiée et considérée au point de vue de la famille et de la société* (Paris: Adrien Delahaye, 1861).

102. Lunier, review of Trélat's *La Folie lucide* in *Amp.* 7 (1861):663–64.

103. *Amp.* 11 (1868):287–89. See also Renaudin, "Observations sur les recherches," p. 496.

104. Berthier, "Des causes de l'encombrement," pp. 368–78.

105. *Amp.* 5 (1865):149. See also L. Delasiauve, "Psychologie educatrice: Lacenaire," *Journal de médecine mentale* 4 (1864):275.

106. See Jan Ellen Goldstein, "French Psychiatry in Social and Political Perspective: The Formation of a New Profession 1820–1860" (Ph.D. diss., Columbia University, 1978), p. 158.

107. Jan Goldstein, "'Moral Contagion': A Professional Ideology of Medicine and Psychiatry in Eighteenth- and Nineteenth-Century France," in Gerald L. Geison, ed., *Professions and the French State, 1700–1900* (Philadelphia: University of Pennsylvania Press, 1984), p. 200 (hereafter cited as Geison, *Professions*).

108. Jacques Donzelot, *The Policing of Families,* trans. Robert Hurley (New York: Pantheon, 1979). See also Jacques Léonard, *La Médecine entre les savoirs et les pouvoirs: Histoire intellectuelle et politique de la médecine française au XIXe siècle* (Paris: Editions Aubier Montaigne, 1982), pp. 161–63.

109. See M. Macario, review of Fr. Devay's *Traité spécial d'hygiène des familles, particulièrement dans ses rapports avec le mariage, au physique et au moral, et les maladies héréditaires* in *Amp.* 5 (1859): 490–95.

110. Cited in Erwin H. Ackerknecht, "Hygiene in France 1815–1848," *Bulletin of the History of Medicine* 22 (1948):117–55.

111. J. Rochard, "L' Influence de l'hygiène sur la grandeur et la prospérité des nations," *Ann. d'hygiène* 13 (1885):20–21.

112. Morel, *Traité,* pp. 77–78, 590, 595.

113. 25 May 1868 meeting of the Société médico-psychologique, *Amp.* 11 (1868):288.

114. Morel, *Traité,* p. 609.

115. Susanna Barrows, "After the Commune: Alcoholism, Temperance, and Literature in the Early Third Republic," in John M. Merriman, ed., *Consciousness and Class Experience in Nineteenth-Century Europe* (New York: Holmes and Meier, 1979), p. 211.

116. Michael R. Marrus, "Social Drinking in the *Belle Epoque,*" *Journal of Social History* 7 (1974):118–19. According to a recent treatment of the history of French temperance, before the turn of the century the Société française de tempérance had been "devoted mainly to talk" and little to action. See Patricia E. Prestwich, *Drink and the Politics of Social Reform: Antialcoholism in France Since 1870* (Palo Alto, Calif.: Society for the Promotion of Science and Scholarship, 1988), p. 66.

117. J. Séglas, "Une famille de dégénérés," 28 Feb. 1887 meeting of the Société médico-psychologique in *Amp.* 5 (1887):473–74.

118. Ch. Féré, "Morbid Heredity," *Popular Science Monthly* 47 (1895):396–97.

119. For an account of the debate over this bill, see Nye, *Crime*, pp. 76–77.

120. E. Billod, "De la conduite à tenir quand on est consulté par un sujet qui se croit menacé de folie parce qu'il est issu de parents aliénés," *Amp.* 9 (1883):424, 426.

121. For a more detailed discussion of medicine's use of science to restore "legitimate complexity," see Paul Starr, *The Social Transformation of American Medicine* (New York: Basic, 1982), pp. 54–59.

122. Séglas, "Une famille de dégénérés," p. 475; see also Ach. Foville, review of *Bulletins et mémoires de la Société d'anthropologie de Paris* in *Amp.* 9 (1867):110–31.

123. Roger Cooter, "Phrenology and British Alienists ca. 1825–1845," in Scull, *Madhouses*, p. 76.

124. Erwin H. Ackerknecht, *Therapeutics: From the Primitives to the Twentieth Century* (New York: Hafner, 1973), p. 3.

Chapter Seven:
Science, Politics, and Psychiatric Hereditarianism
in the Nineteenth Century

1. For Auguste Comte's characterization of the scientist as a moral authority, see Gertrud Lenzer, ed., *Auguste Comte and Positivism: The Essential Writings* (Chicago: University of Chicago Press, 1984), pp. 215–16.

2. Roger Cooter, "Phrenology and British Alienists ca. 1825–1845," in Andrew Scull, ed., *Madhouses, Mad-Doctors, and Madmen: The Social History of Psychiatry in the Victorian Era* (Philadelphia: University of Pennsylvania Press, 1981), p. 67.

3. P. A. Piorry, *De l'hérédité dans les maladies* (Paris: Bury, 1840), pp. 31–32.

4. Ach. Foville, review of J. Moreau de Tours's *La Psychologie morbide dans ses rapports avec la philosophie de l'histoire*, *Amp.* 6 (1860):155.

5. J. Luys, "Des maladies héréditaires" (unpublished medical thesis, Paris, Faculty of Medicine, 1863).

6. H. Grainger-Steward, "De la folie héréditaire," trans E. Dumesnil, *Amp.* 4 (1864):356.

7. E. Dupouy, "Recherches sur les maladies constitutionnelles et diathésiques dans leurs rapports avec les névroses et principalement avec la folie," *Amp.* 8 (1866):24.

8. See Dr. Bourdin, review of A.-J. Gaussail's *De l'influence de l'hé-*

rédité sur la production de la surexcitation nerveuse sur les maladies qui en resultent et des moyens de les guérir in *Amp*. 6 (1845):143–47.

9. E. Gintrac, "Mémoire sur l'influence de l'hérédité sur la production de la surexcitation nerveuse," *Mémoires de l'Académie royale de médecine* 11 (1845):193–382.

10. J. Moreau de Tours, *La Psychologie morbide dans ses rapports avec la philosophie de l'histoire ou de l'influence des névropathies sur le dynamisme intellectuel* (Paris: Masson, 1859).

11. Fernand Levillain, "Charcot et l'école de la Salpêtrière," *Revue encyclopédique* 4 (1894): 108–15.

12. Sigmund Freud, *Collected Papers*, ed. Ernest Jones, trans. Joan Riviere, 6 vols. (London: Hogarth Press, 1956), 1:23.

13. J. Dejerine, *L'Hérédité dans les maladies du système nerveux* (Paris: Asselin et Houzeau, 1886), pp. 28–29.

14. Ch. Féré, "La famille névropathique," *Archives de neurologie* 7 (1884):1–43, 173–91.

15. E. Régis, "Note sur quelques cas de folie héréditaire chez les gens âgés," *Amp*. 5 (1887):224; J. Ramadier and H. Mabille, "Un dégénéré juvenile," ibid., p. 375. See also J. Séglas, "Une famille de dégénérés," ibid., p. 472.

16. L. Landouzy and G. Ballet, "Du rôle de l'hérédité nerveuse dans la genèse de l'ataxie locomotrice progressive," *Amp*. 11 (1884):29–37.

17. For this trend in nineteenth-century psychiatry, see Jan Goldstein, *Console and Classify: The French Psychiatric Profession in the Nineteenth Century* (Cambridge: Cambridge University Press, 1987), pp. 322–38.

18. B. A. Morel, *Traité des dégénérescences physiques, intellectuelles, et morales de l'espèce humaine* (Paris: Baillière, 1857), pp. xiii, 282–83n., 313–14n. (hereafter cited as *Traité*).

19. J. Schiller, "Physiology's Struggle for Independence in the First Half of the Nineteenth Century," *History of Science* 7 (1968):74.

20. C. E. Brown-Séquard, "On the Hereditary Transmission of Effects of Certain Injuries to the Nervous System," *Lancet* 1 (1875):7–8.

21. Ach. Foville, "Recherches cliniques et statistiques sur la transmission héréditaire de l'épilepsie," *Amp*. 11 (1868):205.

22. H. Legrand du Saulle, *La Folie héréditaire: Leçons professées à l'école pratique* (Paris: Adrien Delahaye, 1873), p. 15. See also Ch. Féré, "La famille névropathique," p. 5.

23. Robert A. Nye, *Crime, Madness, and Politics in Modern France: The Medical Concept of National Decline* (Princeton: Princeton University Press, 1984), pp. 119–21.

24. Dr. Campagne, "Manie raisonnante: Etiologie et pathogénie," *Amp.* 12 (1868):1–34, 207–34.

25. Ibid., p. 3.

26. Th. Ribot, *Heredity: A Psychological Study of its Phenomena, Laws, Causes, and Consequences* (New York: Appleton, 1875), p. 391 (hereafter cited as Ribot, *Heredity*).

27. L. Delasiauve, "Quelques mots sur l'hérédité morbide, par M. A. Mitivié," *Journal de médecine mentale* 2 (1862):97.

28. H. Grainger-Steward, "De la folie héréditaire," pp. 356–57.

29. J. Baillarger, "A Course of Lectures on the Diseases of the Brain and Insanity; Delivered at the Salpêtrière, Paris," *Lancet* 1 (1845):313.

30. *Amp.* 11 (1868):273.

31. *Amp.* 9 (1883):419–32.

32. Léonard, *La Médecine entre les savoirs et les pouvoirs: Histoire intellectuelle et politique de la médecine française au XIXe siècle* (Paris: Editions Aubier Montaigne, 1982), p. 153.

33. For medical reviews of this literature, see Dr. Fonssagrives, *Annales d'hygiène publique et de médecine légale* 19 (1863):467–70 (hereafter cited as *Ann. d'hygiène*); J. Falret, "De la consanguinité," *Archives générales de médecine* 5 (1865):209–17, 464–80; see also Dr. Boudin, "Dangers des unions consanguines," *Ann. d'hygiène* 18 (1862): 5–82.

34. G. Lagneau, "Etude de statistique anthropologique sur la population parisienne," *Ann. d'hygiène* 32 (1869):249–79.

35. Nye, *Crime*, p. 141

36. See for example, A. E. Carter, *The Idea of Decadence in French Literature* (Toronto: University of Toronto Press, 1958); Eric C. Hansen, *Disaffection and Decadence: A Crisis in French Intellectual Thought 1848–1898* (Washington, D.C.: University Press of America, 1982); Koenraad W. Swart, *The Sense of Decadence in Nineteenth-Century France* (The Hague: Nijhoff, 1964).

37. Charles de Remusat, "Du Pessimisme politique," *Revue des deux mondes* 28 (1860):729. Cited in Daniel Pick, *Faces of Degeneration: A European Disorder, c.1848–c.1918* (Cambridge: Cambridge University Press, 1989), pp. 56–57. For more on the political crisis of confidence in France after 1848, see ibid., pp. 37–106. Pick's book, a brilliant exercise in intellectual history, and Nye's pioneering *Crime, Madness, and Politics* are the best accounts of French cultural and social interest in decadence and degeneration.

38. Susanna Barrows, "After the Commune: Alcoholism, Temperance, and Literature in the Early Third Republic," in John M. Merriman, ed., *Consciousness and Class Experience in Nineteenth-Century Europe* (New York: Holmes and Meier, 1979), p. 208.

39. Jean Borie, *Mythologies de l'hérédité au XIXe siècle* (Paris: Editions galilées, 1981), p. 180.

40. Cl. Digeon, *La Crise allemande de la pensée française (1870–1914)* (Paris: Presses universitaires de France, 1959), pp. 328–29.

41. Nye, *Crime*, pp. 54–55.

42. Ibid., p. 54.

43. For the nationalist revival of 1905–1914, see Eugen Weber, *The Nationalist Revival in France 1905–1914* (Berkeley and Los Angeles: University of California Press, 1968).

44. Digeon, *La Crise allemande*, p. 353.

45. For example, see Swart, *Sense* and Carter, *Idea of Decadence*.

46. See Nye, *Crime*, p. 133.

47. Jan Goldstein, "'Moral Contagion': A Professional Ideology of Medicine and Psychiatry in Eighteenth- and Nineteenth-Century France," in Gerald L. Geison, ed., *Professions and the French State, 1700–1900* (Philadelphia: University of Pennsylvania Press, 1984), pp. 205–11.

48. Prosper Lucas, *Traité philosophique et physiologique de l'hérédité naturelle dans les états de santé et de maladie du système nerveux*, 2 vols. (Paris: Baillière, 1847–1850), 1:1–6. See also Jean Borie, *Mythologies de l'hérédité*, pp. 13, 69–73.

49. L. F. E. Renaudin, "Observations sur les recherches statistiques relative à l'aliénation mentale," *Amp.* 2 (1856):356–57; Moreau, *La Psychologie morbide*, p. 77.

50. Cited in Ribot, *Heredity*, p. 87.

51. U. Trélat, *La Folie lucide etudiée au point de vue de la famille et de la société* (Paris: Adrien Delahaye, 1861), pp. 6–11, 317–25.

52. J. V. Laborde, *Les Hommes et les actes de l'insurrection de Paris devant la psychologie morbide: Lettres à M. le docteur Moreau (de Tours)* (Paris: Germer-Baillière, 1872), pp. iii, 2–3.

53. Ibid., p. 89.

54. *Amp.* 7 (1872):257.

55. *Amp.* 6 (1871):222–41.

56. H. Taguet, "De l'hérédité dans l'alcoolisme," *Amp.* 18 (1877): 5–17.

57. *Amp.* 6 (1871):222–41.

58. Pick, *Faces of Degeneration*, p. 53.

59. Charles E. Rosenberg, *No Other Gods: On Science and American Social Thought* (Baltimore: Johns Hopkins University Press, 1976), chap. 1, "The Bitter Fruit: Heredity, Disease, and Social Thought in Nineteenth-Century America," pp. 25–53.

60. Barrows, "After the Commune," p. 209.

61. Nye, *Crime*, p. 170.

62. Ibid., pp. 231–32.

63. Ibid., p. 50.

64. Robert Locke, *French Legitimists and the Politics of Moral Order in the Early Third Republic* (Princeton: Princeton University Press, 1974), pp. 176–77. Cited in Nye, *Crime*, p. 72.

65. Ibid., p. 68.

66. Ruth Harris has argued that psychiatrists in France, while often relying on the theory of hereditary degeneracy and neurophysiological involuntarism, "were as obsessed by the question of moral agency as jurists" and "believed in the possibility of promoting the autonomy of the individual." See Ruth Harris, *Murders and Madness: Medicine, Law, and Society in the Fin-de-Siècle* (Oxford: Oxford University Press, 1989), p. 322.

67. Morel, *Traité*, p. 5.

68. Nye, *Crime*, p. 126.

69. Theodore M. Brown, "The Rise of Baconianism in Seventeenth Century England," in *Science and History: Studies in Honour of Edward Rosen* (Warsaw: Polish Academy of Sciences, 1978), pp. 501–22; see also idem, "The College of Physicians and the Acceptance of Iatromechanism in England, 1665–1695," *Bulletin of the History of Medicine* 44 (1970):12–30.

70. There is a substantial literature on the cultural importance of science in nineteenth-century England and America. For a recent and excellent bibliography of this literature, see S. E. D. Shortt, *Victorian Lunacy: Richard M. Bucke and the Practice of Late Nineteenth-Century Psychiatry* (Cambridge: Cambridge University Press, 1986), especially pp. 186–87. See also idem, "Physicians, Science, and Status: Issues in the Professionalization of Anglo-American Medicine in the Nineteenth Century," *Medical History* 27 (1983): 51–68.

71. Sanford Elwitt, *The Making of the Third Republic: Class and Politics in France 1868–1884* (Baton Rouge: Louisiana State University Press, 1975), pp. 170–229.

Conclusion:
The Social History of Psychiatric Knowledge

1. Georges Genil-Perrin, *Histoire des origines et de l'évolution de l'idée de dégénérescence en médecine mentale* (Paris: Leclerc, 1913), p. 9.

2. Ibid., pp. 273–75. For other psychiatric accounts that echoed Genil-Perrin's criticism, see V. Demole, "Considérations biologiques sur l'hérédité dans les maladies mentales," *Annales médico-psychologiques* 5

(1914):417–31; and E. Toulouse and M. Mignard, "La Théorie confusionnelle et l'auto-conduction," ibid., pp. 641–57.

3. Henri F. Ellenberger, *The Discovery of the Unconscious: The History and Evolution of Dynamic Psychiatry* (New York: Basic Books, 1970).

4. Etienne Trillat, "Une histoire de la psychiatrie au XXe siècle," in Jacques Postel and Claude Quétel, eds., *Nouvelle histoire de la psychiatrie* (Toulouse: Privat, 1983), pp. 453–79.

5. Richard W. Fox, *So Far Disordered in Mind: Insanity in California 1870–1930* (Berkeley, Los Angeles, and London: University of California Press, 1978), pp. 167–74.

6. For similar developments in Anglo-American psychiatry, see S. E. D. Shortt, *Victorian Lunacy: Richard M. Bucke and the Practice of Late Nineteenth-Century Psychiatry* (Cambridge: Cambridge University Press, 1986), pp. 108–109. For a psychiatric admission that the poor were more disposed to mental alienation than were the affluent classes, see P. Naecke, "La Valeur des signes de dégénérescence dans l'étude des maladies mentales," *Annales médico-psychologiques* 22 (1894):259 (hereafter cited as *Amp.*).

7. H. Damaye, "La Psychiatrie actuelle et la thérapeutique des affections curables," *Amp.* 3 (1913):290–98.

8. See Robert A. Nye, *Crime, Madness, and Politics in Modern France: The Medical Concept of National Decline* (Princeton: Princeton University Press, 1984), pp. 310–29. The term "nationalist revival" is borrowed from Eugen Weber, *The Nationalist Revival in France, 1905–1914* (Berkeley: University of California Press, 1959). See also idem, "Gymnastics and Sports in *Fin-de-Siècle* France: Opium of the Classes?" *American Historical Review* 76 (1971):70–99; "Pierre de Coubertin and the Introduction of Organized Sport in France," *Journal of Contemporary History* 5 (1970):3–26. For an account of the distinctive features of French eugenics, see William Schneider, "Toward the Improvement of the Human Race: The History of Eugenics in France," *Journal of Modern History* 54 (1982):268–91.

9. John Eros, "The Positivist Generation of French Republicanism," *Sociological Review* 3 (1955):255–77. See also Sanford Elwitt, *The Making of the Third Republic: Class and Politics in France 1868–1884* (Baton Rouge: Louisiana State University Press, 1975), pp. 171–229; William R. Keylor, "Anti-Clericalism and Educational Reform in the French Third Republic: A Retrospective Evaluation," *History of Education Quarterly* 21 (1983):95–103.

10. Theodore Zeldin, *France 1848–1945: Politics and Anger* (Oxford: Oxford University Press, 1979), pp. 276–318. For an informative discussion of solidarism and its implications for state social welfare, see Judith F.

Stone, *The Search for Social Peace: Reform Legislation in France, 1890–1914* (Albany: State University of New York Press, 1985), especially chaps. 5 and 6.

11. See Andrew Scull, *Decarceration: Community Treatment and the Deviant: A Radical View* (Englewood Cliffs, N. J.: Prentice-Hall, 1977).

12. Ian Dowbiggin, "French Psychiatry, Hereditarianism, and Professional Legitimacy, 1840–1900," in Andrew T. Scull and Steven Spitzer, eds., *Research in Law, Deviance and Social Control* 7 (1985):135–65.

13. See Thomas S. Kuhn, *The Structure of Scientific Revolutions*, 2nd ed. (Chicago: University of Chicago Press, 1970).

14. Carl F. Kaestle, "Social Reform and the Urban School," *History of Education Quarterly* 12 (1972):218.

15. Peter McCandless, "Liberty and Lunacy: The Victorians and Wrongful Confinement," in Andrew T. Scull, ed., *Madhouses, Mad-Doctors, and Madmen: The Social History of Psychiatry in the Victorian Era* (Philadelphia: University of Pennsylvania Press, 1981), pp. 339–62.

16. Nancy Tomes, *A Generous Confidence: Thomas Story Kirkbride and the Art of Asylum-Keeping 1840–1883* (Cambridge: Cambridge University Press, 1984), pp. 222–63.

17. Julie V. Brown, "A Sociohistorical Perspective on Deinstitutionalization: The Case of Late Imperial Russia," in Scull and Spitzer, eds., *Research in Law, Deviance, and Social Control* 7 (1985):167–88.

18. For similar observations, see Stephen J. Kunitz, "The Historical Roots and Ideological Functions of Disease Concepts in Three Primary Care Specialties," *Bulletin of the History of Medicine* 57 (1983):412–32.

19. Steven Spitzer and Andrew Scull, Introduction to Scull and Spitzer, eds., *Research in Law, Deviance, and Social Control* 7 (1985):11.

20. For the history of prefrontal lobotomies, see Elliot S. Valenstein's *Great and Desperate Cures: The Rise and Decline of Psychosurgery and Other Radical Treatments for Mental Illness* (New York: Basic, 1986). See also Andrew Scull's "Desperate Remedies: A Gothic Tale of Madness and Modern Medicine," *Psychological Medicine* 17 (1987):561–77.

21. Paul Starr, *The Social Transformation of American Medicine* (New York: Basic, 1982), pp. 54–59.

22. For the lack of interest among U.S. superintendents in theoretical issues, see John Pitts, "The Association of Medical Superintendents of American Institutions for the Insane, 1844–1892: A Case of Specialism in American Medicine," (Ph.D. diss., University of Pennsylvania, 1979), especially pp. 29–30.

23. For the 1881–1885 "crisis of professional legitimacy" in American psychiatry, see Pitts, ibid., chap. 7; see also Gerald N. Grob, *Mental Illness and American Society, 1875–1940* (Princeton: Princeton University Press, 1983), pp. 69–71.

24. Charles E. Rosenberg, "The Crisis in Psychiatric Legitimacy: Reflections on Psychiatry, Medicine, and Public Policy," in G. Kriegman, R. D. Gardner, D. W. Abse, eds., *American Psychiatry: Past, Present, and Future* (Charlottesville: University Press of Virginia, 1975), p. 146.

25. Gerald N. Grob, "Rediscovering Asylums: The Unhistorical History of the Mental Hospital," in Morris J. Vogel and Charles E. Rosenberg, eds., *The Therapeutic Revolution: Essays in the Social History of American Medicine* (Philadelphia: University of Pennsylvania Press, 1979), pp. 151–52. See also idem, *Mental Illness and American Society 1875–1940* (Princeton: Princeton University Press, 1983), pp. 120–22.

26. Stephen J. Kunitz, "The Historical Roots and Ideological Functions of Disease Concepts in Three Primary Care Specialties," pp. 413–14.

27. Some of the most important works of Michel Foucault include *Madness and Civilization: A History of Insanity in the Age of Reason* (New York: Pantheon, 1965), *Discipline and Punish: The Birth of the Prison* (New York: Pantheon, 1977), *Power/Knowledge: Selected Interviews and Other Writings, 1972–1977* (London: Harvester, 1980). For Foucault's use of the term "docile bodies," see *Discipline and Punish,* pp. 135–69. For insightful discussions of Foucault's contributions to the historiography of psychiatry, see Daniel Pick, *Faces of Degeneration: A European Disorder, c.1848–c.1918* (Cambridge: Cambridge University Press, 1989), pp. 43–44, 235–37; Andrew Scull, *Social Order/Mental Disorder: Anglo-American Psychiatry in Historical Perspective* (Berkeley: University of California Press, 1989), pp. 13–20. For the "professional imperialism of the psychiatrists" in nineteenth-century France, see Jan Goldstein, *Console and Classify: The French Psychiatric Profession in the Nineteenth Century* (Cambridge: Cambridge University Press, 1987), especially p. 333.

28. Rosenberg, "The Crisis in Psychiatric Legitimacy," p. 135.

29. For an astute analysis of psychiatry's present-day problems and their influence on the recent move to a more biological understanding of mental illness, see Michael J. Bader, "Is Psychiatry Going Out of Its Mind?" *Tikkun* 4 (1989):43–48.

30. For example, see Paul S. Appelbaum, "Crazy in the Streets," *Commentary* 38 (1987):34–39. I am indebted to Wilfred M. McClay for this reference.

31. See especially Christopher Lasch, *The Culture of Narcissism: American Life in An Age of Diminishing Expectations* (New York: Norton, 1978).

Index

Compositor: Interactive Composition Corporation
Text: 11/13 Caledonia
Display: Caledonia

WITHDRAWN

No longer the property of the
Boston Public Library.
Sale of this material benefits the Library